Michelle

VOCALLY DISRUPTIVE BEHAVIOUR (VDB)

Michelle Todoruk-Orchard

VOCALLY DISRUPTIVE BEHAVIOUR (VDB) IN THE OLDER ADULT WITH DEMENTIA

Theories and Strategies to assist Families and Staff. Understand VDB in Older Adults with Dementia Living in Long Term Care

VDM Verlag Dr. Müller

Impressum/Imprint (nur für Deutschland/ only for Germany)
Bibliografische Information der Deutschen Nationalbibliothek: Die Deutsche Nationalbibliothek verzeichnet diese Publikation in der Deutschen Nationalbibliografie; detaillierte bibliografische Daten sind im Internet über http://dnb.d-nb.de abrufbar.

Alle in diesem Buch genannten Marken und Produktnamen unterliegen warenzeichen-, marken- oder patentrechtlichem Schutz bzw. sind Warenzeichen oder eingetragene Warenzeichen der jeweiligen Inhaber. Die Wiedergabe von Marken, Produktnamen, Gebrauchsnamen, Handelsnamen, Warenbezeichnungen u.s.w. in diesem Werk berechtigt auch ohne besondere Kennzeichnung nicht zu der Annahme, dass solche Namen im Sinne der Warenzeichen- und Markenschutzgesetzgebung als frei zu betrachten wären und daher von jedermann benutzt werden dürften.

Coverbild: www.purestockx.com

Verlag: VDM Verlag Dr. Müller Aktiengesellschaft & Co. KG
Dudweiler Landstr. 99, 66123 Saarbrücken, Deutschland
Telefon +49 681 9100-698, Telefax +49 681 9100-988, Email: info@vdm-verlag.de

Herstellung in Deutschland:
Schaltungsdienst Lange o.H.G., Berlin
Books on Demand GmbH, Norderstedt
Reha GmbH, Saarbrücken
Amazon Distribution GmbH, Leipzig
ISBN: 978-3-639-16073-4

Imprint (only for USA, GB)
Bibliographic information published by the Deutsche Nationalbibliothek: The Deutsche Nationalbibliothek lists this publication in the Deutsche Nationalbibliografie; detailed bibliographic data are available in the Internet at http://dnb.d-nb.de .
Any brand names and product names mentioned in this book are subject to trademark, brand or patent protection and are trademarks or registered trademarks of their respective holders. The use of brand names, product names, common names, trade names, product descriptions etc. even without a particular marking in this works is in no way to be construed to mean that such names may be regarded as unrestricted in respect of trademark and brand protection legislation and could thus be used by anyone.

Cover image: www.purestockx.com

Publisher:
VDM Verlag Dr. Müller Aktiengesellschaft & Co. KG
Dudweiler Landstr. 99, 66123 Saarbrücken, Germany
Phone +49 681 9100-698, Fax +49 681 9100-988, Email: info@vdm-publishing.com

Copyright © 2010 by the author and VDM Verlag Dr. Müller Aktiengesellschaft & Co. KG and licensors
All rights reserved. Saarbrücken 2010

Printed in the U.S.A.
Printed in the U.K. by (see last page)
ISBN: 978-3-639-16073-4

ACKNOWLEDGEMENTS

I would like to thank the Informal Caregiver Participants and
The Staff at Deer Lodge and Riverview Health Centre

DEDICATION

I would like to dedicate this practicum to my wonderful husband, Gerry Orchard.
He has been a constant source of strength and support.

VOCALLY DISRUPTIVE BEHAVIOUR IN THE OLDER ADULT WITH DEMENTIA

CHAPTER 1: Statement of the Problem
    1.1 Introduction/Background of the problem 5
    1.2 Statement/Significance of the problem 6
    1.3 Purpose and Goals of the practicum 7

CHAPTER 2: Conceptual Framework 8

CHAPTER 3: Review of the Literature
    3.1   Overview of Vocally Disruptive Behaviours 14
        3.1.1 Historical Perspectives of Vocally Disruptive Behaviour 14
        3.1.2 Theoretical perspectives 17
        3.1.3 Definitions 21
        3.1.4 Prevalence 23
        3.1.5 Profile of the vocally disruptive resident 24
    3.2 Assessment and Management Interventions 28
        3.2.1 Assessment 28
        3.2.2 Management Interventions 31
    3.3 Overview of Research Studies 33
        3.3.1 Types of studies 33
        3.3.2 Location of studies 34
        3.3.3 Methodologies 34
        3.3.4 Comparability and generalizability of results 38
    3.4 Gaps in the literature 38

CHAPTER 4: Design of the Practicum
    4.1 Design of practicum project 41
    4.2 Definitions 41
    4.3 The setting 43
    4.4 The participants...44
    4.5 Information gathering and evaluation methods 45
    4.6 Ethical considerations 46

CHAPTER 5: The Conduct of the Practicum
    5.1 Demographic characteristics 48
    5.2 Results of Initial Assessment 50
    5.3 Analysis of Initial Interview and Development of Interventions 54
    5.4 Results of Educational Sessions 57
    5.5 Follow-up Telephone Call 58
    5.6 The Focus Group 59

CHAPTER 6: Discussions and Conclusions
    6.1 Discussion, Evaluation, Recommendations and Conclusion 63
    6.2 Limitations 65
    6.3 Future directions 65

References 66

Appendices
    Appendix A: The Calgary Family Assessment Model – Interview Guide 71
    Appendix B: The Calgary Family Intervention Model 77
    Appendix C: Demographic Information 78
    Appendix D: Focus Group Questions..79
    Appendix E: Information sheet for staff/MDT 81
    Appendix F: Information sheet for PCM/CNS to read to potential participants ...83
    Appendix G: Consent Form and Information on Participation............................85
    Appendix H: Understanding Vocally Disruptive Behaviours for Family and
                   Informal Caregivers 90
    Appendix I: Revised Education Package for Family and Informal Caregivers 97
    Appendix J: Understanding Vocally Disruptive Behaviour for Staff.................. 103

CHAPTER 1: STATEMENT OF THE PROBLEM

Introduction/ Background of the Problem

As the elderly population in our society continues to increase, the number of older adults that are cognitively impaired due to dementia will also continue to increase (Burgener, Jirovec, Murrell, & Barton, 1992; Finkel, Lyons, & Anderson, 1993; Rossby, Beck, & Heacock,1992). Dementia in older adults is generally progressive in nature and is most often a result of Alzheimer's disease. Due to the progressive nature of dementia, as well as the magnitude of care needs and associated behaviours, institutionalization is often inevitable, as family/informal caregivers are unable to continue to manage care in the community (Buckwalter, Maas, & Reed,1997; Maas, Buckwalter, Kelley, & Stolley,1991; Teri & Lodgson, 1990).

Providing care to the cognitively impaired older adult, whether it be in the community or in a long term care setting is a major challenge for both formal and informal caregivers (Finkel et al., 1993). This challenge can become an even more significant problem when the cognitively impaired resident exhibits disruptive, agitated or aggressive behaviours (Beck & Shue, 1994; Weinrich, Egbert, Eleazer, & Haddock, 1995). Disruptive behaviour occurs frequently in the cognitively impaired older adult as the dementing illness progresses. Research has shown that the prevalence of disruptive behaviour in this group of older adults can range from 24 % to as high as 93% (Beck et al, 1994; Burgio, Jones, Butler, & Engel, 1988; Cohen-Mansfield, Marx, & Rosenthal, 1989; Zimmer, Watson, & Treat, 1984). Often, it is the occurrence of disruptive behaviour that precipitates the family caregiver's decision to move the older adult to a long term care setting (Cohen-Mansfield, 1986; Teri, Larson, & Reifler, 1988; Teri et al., 1990).

Once the decision for admission to long term care has been made, family caregivers may experience difficulty in adjusting to their changing role (Buckwalter et al., 1997; Maas et al., 1990). Turning over care to staff members, learning institutional routines, learning how to visit as well as observing some of the behaviours displayed by their relative can be stressful for family caregivers and can cause conflict with the institutional staff.

Of all the behaviour identified as disruptive, agitated or aggressive, vocally disruptive behaviour (VDB) has been identified as one of the most stressful and frustrating for staff, other residents and family caregivers (Bourgeois, Burgio, Schulz, Beach, & Palmer, 1997; Hallberg, Norberg, & Erikson, 1990; White, Merrie, & Richie, 1996). Family members may find the VDB stressful to a point where they visit less frequently and/or criticize staff for their inability to meet the resident's needs and therefore prevent the disruptive vocalization (Sloane et al., 1997).

Statement/ Significance of the Problem

Although numerous research studies have focused on the experience of informal caregivers of relatives with dementia in the community, relatively little research has been conducted examining informal caregivers' knowledge, perceptions and their relationship with their relative and staff following admission to a long term care facility (Buckwalter et al., 1997; Maas et al., 1990). Health care professionals, most often nurses, have the greatest contact with family caregivers and play a critical role in providing care and support to the resident and family caregiver unit. Family caregivers are among the most important resources for developing the plan of care for the resident. Their involvement is essential to helping nursing staff understand and attempt to manage the vocally disruptive behaviour in the resident with dementia (Scott, 1991). Nurses and other members of the health care team need to know more about family members' perceptions so they can more effectively intervene to ease the stress and burden the family may be experiencing as well as facilitate adjustment and continued involvement of the family caregiver (Maas et al., 1991). Working closely with the family caregivers to increase their knowledge of their family member's vocally disruptive behaviour and understanding their perceptions of the approaches implemented by staff is essential to ultimately providing the highest quality of care and quality of life to the resident with dementia.

Purpose and Goals of the Practicum

The purpose of the practicum was to develop, conduct and evaluate a teaching and support program for informal caregivers of vocally disruptive residents living in a long term care setting. The teaching and support program was based on an individual assessment of each informal caregivers' level of knowledge and their perceptions of the vocally disruptive behaviour of their family member. Evaluation of the program was completed with the informal caregivers in a focus group. Modifications were made to the program based on the evaluative feedback provided by the informal caregivers.

The goals of the practicum were;

1. To assess the knowledge held by informal caregivers of the vocally disruptive behaviour displayed by their family/friend in a long term care setting in the areas of awareness of causes and contributing factors, ability to control the behaviour and staff approaches and management of the VDB,
2. To assess the perceptions held by the informal caregivers of the vocally disruptive behaviour displayed by their family/friend in a long term care setting
3. To prepare and provide an educational and support program for the informal caregivers based on the results of the assessment,
4. To evaluate the teaching and support program with the informal caregivers following completion of the program, and
5. To revise the program based on the evaluative feedback provided by the informal caregivers.

After completion of the practicum, the family teaching and support package will be provided to the two long term care facilities to use in the future. In addition, although not part of the practicum, an educational session regarding vocally disruptive behaviour will be offered for staff at the two facilities to serve as a framework for staff education.

CHAPTER 2: CONCEPTUAL FRAMEWORK

A variety of conceptual frameworks have been adopted by clinicians and researchers to study family members and informal caregivers knowledge, perception, stress levels and coping when caring for a loved one who has been diagnosed with dementia. Frameworks can be grouped into three categories; environmental, stress and coping and family theory.

Betty Neuman (1990) conceptualized a health systems model that focuses on the interaction of the person and environment. Her model describes an open system with major components of stressors, reaction to stressors and the person interacting with the environment. Stressors can occur outside the system, between one or more individuals within the system and within the individual. The individual's reaction to the stressor(s) will be influenced by a number of factors including number and strength of stressors, the length of the encounter with them and their specific meaning to the system as well as past coping skills. Neuman's systems model views families as having both a composite identity and an individual member profile (Neuman, 1989). Although Neuman's model has been used in a variety of clinical settings, one limitation is that it has been applied inconsistently and components of it have been defined differently by various nurse clinicians and researchers.

Lazarus and Folkman (1984) developed a model of Stress, Appraisal and Coping that also emphasized the relationship between the person and environment taking into account the individual characteristics of the person as well as the nature of the event occurring within an environmental context. They postulated that people differ in their sensitivity and vulnerability to certain types of events as well as in their interpretations and reactions to the events. Coping, as defined by Lazarus and Folkman consists of constantly changing cognitive and behavioural efforts to manage specific internal and external demands that are appraised as stressful or exceeding the resources of the person. Lazarus and Folkman's model of stress, appraisal and coping has been applied to a variety of health research examining family members stress and coping patterns both in community and institutional settings. It addresses the individual person rather than the family system and examines stress, appraisal and coping rather than knowledge and perceptions.

More recently, as the study of family systems has received greater attention, several frameworks have evolved that focus less on the family members' reactions to specific behaviours and more on the dynamics of the family system as a whole. McCubbin and McCubbin (1993) developed a family systems model called the Resiliency Model to describe family stress, adjustment and adaptation. The model was designed to assist health professionals in assessing family functioning and intervening in the family system to facilitate both family adjustment and adaptation. The model facilitates assessment of the family system's reaction to the situation or illness and assists the health care professional to develop strategies to evaluate family functioning under stress. This complex framework has been used to work with families in a variety of acute and chronic illness settings. Although it provides a family systems assessment framework, it lacks incorporation of factors that influence intervention.

One of the family systems models that has received wide recognition since its introduction in 1994 is the Calgary Family Assessment Model (CFAM) (Fig. 1) and the Calgary Family Intervention Model (CFIM) (Fig 2). Wright and Leahey (1994) introduced this integrated, multi-dimensional framework that is based on systems theory, cybernetics, communication theory and change theory. This model has been used extensively in a variety of community and institutional settings in working with families dealing with chronic illness, psychosocial problems and life threatening illness (Wright & Leahey, 1994).

The CFAM framework consists of three major categories for assessment and intervention:

"**Structural** – examination of family membership, the relationship among family members and to those outside the family, and the context of the family.

Developmental - examination of the developmental life cycle of the family, tasks to be accomplished and how they are affected by an acute or chronic illness in the family.

Functional - examination of roles and rituals, communication patterns and problem solving" (Wright & Leahey, 1994 pp 37.).

Each of the three categories contains several sub-categories. The nurse decides which sub-categories are relevant and appropriate to utilize with each family at each point in time (Wright & Leahey, 1994). For the purposes of the practicum the first and third categories, structural and functional, will be utilized. In the structural category, parts of two sub-categories will be examined with each informal caregiver and are indicated in bold type (Fig. 1). The functional expressive assessment will include examination of communication patterns, roles, influences, beliefs and alliances. In terms of developmental stage, all caregiver participants in the practicum are in the stage of families later in life.

Figure 1 - The Calgary Family Assessment Model

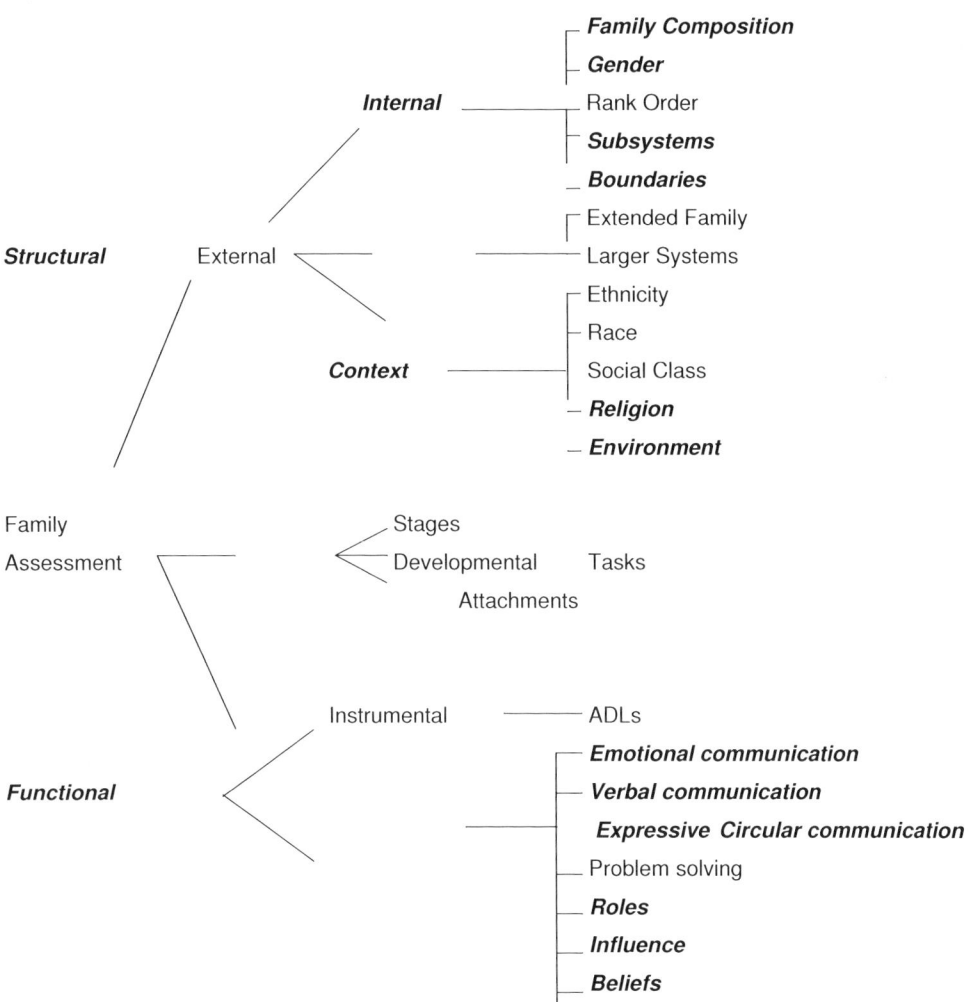

Once assessment is completed using the CFAM, the nurse is able to develop interventions based on the framework of the Calgary Family Intervention Model (CFIM). The Calgary Family Intervention Model is a companion model to the Calgary Family Assessment Model. CFIM "is an organizing framework for conceptualizing the intersection between a particular domain of family functioning and the specific intervention offered by the nurse. CFIM (Figure 2) is focused on promoting, improving, and/or sustaining effective family functioning in three domains: cognitive, affective and behavioural" (Wright & Leahey, 1994, p.99).

Figure 2- The Calgary Family Intervention Model (CFIM)

		Interventions Offered By Nurse
Domains of Cognitive Family Functioning	Affective	
	Behavioural	Fit" or Effectiveness

Interventions in the cognitive domain include commending family and individual strengths, offering information/opinions, reframing and offering education. Interventions in the affective domain include validating/normalizing emotional responses, storying the illness experience, and drawing forth family support. Interventions targeted at changing the behavioural domain include encouraging family members to be caregivers, encouraging respite, and devising rituals. Interventions can be in individual or multiple domains and can be as simple or complex as the nurse assesses appropriate for the family and the situation. Any interventions should be directed toward achieving goals that have been developed with the nurse and family as partners (Wright & Leahey, 1994). The ultimate goal is to assist families to develop new ways of coping and problem solving when faced with an acute or chronic health situation. For this practicum the student developed interventions for informal caregivers in the cognitive, affective and/or behavioural domain as indicated based on their individual assessments.

The Calgary Family Assessment and Intervention Models was utilized as the conceptual framework for this practicum. The CFAM provided a comprehensive assessment framework that assisted the student in interviewing and assessing each informal caregiver's knowledge and perception of their experience with a vocally disruptive relative who is a resident in a long term care facility. Furthermore, the CFIM guided the student in the development of interventions targeted at the appropriate domain(s) for each informal caregiver.

CHAPTER 3: REVIEW OF THE LITERATURE
Overview of Vocally Disruptive Behaviour (VDB)

Thirty seven articles were found in the literature related to vocally disruptive behaviour in older adults living in long term care. This literature was reviewed from a historical perspective. Two major theoretical perspectives were examined in relation to causes and contributing factors. Definitions, prevalence and a profile of the vocally disruptive resident are presented. Assessment and management literature is reviewed and discussed. Research studies presented in the literature are examined in relation to type of research and scientific rigor, location of studies and methodologies as well as comparability and generalizability of results. Finally, gaps in the literature are discussed, specifically highlighting the significance of the family caregiver's perspective and involvement in care of the vocally disruptive older adult in a long term care setting.

Historical Perspectives

Vocally Disruptive Behaviour (VDB) in older adults in personal care home settings have existed for as many years as institutionalized care has existed. In the 1960's and 1970's it appears that little or no attention was devoted to the study of vocally disruptive behaviour. This is evidenced by a lack of literature on this topic spanning this 20 year period. It wasn't until the early 1980's that vocally disruptive behaviour began to receive consistent attention from clinicians and researchers from the nursing, allied health and medical professions. Although reasons for the rapidly growing interest are not specifically addressed in the literature, all behaviour considered as disruptive, agitated or aggressive in older adults began to receive attention in research studies (Beck et al, 1994; Burgio et al., 1988; Cohen-Mansfield et al., 1989, 1990, 1992; Hallberg et al., 1990; Finkel et al., 1993;; Weinrich et al., 1995; Zimmer et al, 1984).

Articles related specifically to VDB began to appear in the early 1980's (Zachow, 1984). Much of this early literature provided case study descriptions of vocally disruptive behaviour in individual patients or residents and a description of interventions introduced on a trial and error basis in attempts to decrease the individual's vocally disruptive behaviour (Christie, & Ferguson, 1988; Zachow, 1984). Other early literature included chapters in medical textbooks attempting to describe reasons for the occurrence of vocally disruptive behaviour (often labeled as screaming and shouting) and approaches to management (Stokes, 1988). This literature, although not research based, provided a beginning attempt to define vocally disruptive behaviour. The concept of individualized assessment and interventions as well as a multi-disciplinary team approach to assessment and care were introduced.

Actual research studies examining vocally disruptive behaviour, both quantitative and qualitative, began to appear in the late 1980's and early 1990's in a number of countries. One of the earliest research studies examining 'noise making' amongst the elderly in long term care was conducted in Canada at the Sunnybrook Hospital in Toronto by Ryan, Tainsh, Kolodny, Lendrum, and Fisher, in 1988. This early work examined the prevalence of vocally disruptive behaviour and provided one of the first broad definitions of VDB that would be used by future researchers.

In Sweden, Ingeborg Hallberg and colleagues (1990) began a series of qualitative and quantitative studies examining vocally disruptive patients in psychogeriatric wards. This Swedish study was aimed at identifying patterns or clusters of functional impairment in vocally disruptive patients (Hallberg, Norberg, & Erikson, 1990). Subsequent studies conducted in Sweden by Hallberg and associates examined various aspects of VDB including attempting to provide a thorough description of vocally disruptive behaviour in regards to amount, level, duration, content and type (Hallberg, Edberg, Nordmark, Johnsson, & Norberg, 1993), as well as studies examining staff perspective (Hallberg, & Norberg, 1990), differences in care provided (Hallberg et al, 1990; Hallberg, Norberg & Johnsson,1993), and the relationship to previous personality traits (Holst, Hallberg, & Gustavson, 1997).

In the same year in the USA, research efforts began to focus on VDB. From 1986-1990, Jiska Cohen-Mansfield and colleagues were pioneers responsible for defining and researching behaviour described as agitated, aggressive and disruptive in older adults living in a nursing home setting. In 1990, they examined the reported prevalence of vocally disruptive behaviour and its existing definitions. The aim of this early study was to develop an overall picture of the characteristics of a resident with vocally disruptive behaviour. This research began to study the link between VDB and personal characteristics and care needs of the resident. At the same time it began to identify potential links to the environment. Cohen-Mansfield and colleagues introduced standardized reliable and valid measurement tools for the study of vocally disruptive behaviour at this time (Cohen-Mansfield, Werner, & Marx, 1990).

In the USA, Cariaga and associates were also beginning to study vocally disruptive behaviour among geriatric residents in nursing homes. In 1991, they examined the prevalence, frequency, duration and typology of vocally disruptive behaviour, adding to the growing body of literature on this subject (Cariaga, Burgio, Flynn, & Martin, 1991).

Over the next ten years researchers continued to examine various aspects of vocally disruptive behaviour. Many articles written during this time frame were based on research studies that examined a wide variety of inter-related topics: staff attitudes and feelings (Whall, Gillis, Yankou, Booth, & Beel-Bates, 1992); relationship to sundown syndrome (Wallace, 1994); assessment and management of vocally disruptive behaviours (Beck et al., 1998; Sloane, Davidson, Knight, Tangen, & Mitchell 1999); implementation and evaluation of interventions (Burgio, 1997; Burgio, Scilley, & Hardin, 1996; Casby, & Holm,1994; Cohen-Mansfield, Marx, & Werner, 1992; Rantz, 1994) and the use of computer technology to assist research (Burgio, 1997; Yurick, Burgio, & Paton, 1995). Other articles provided an overview of knowledge on the subject to date or provided opinions (not research based) related to various assessment and management options (Carlyle, Killick, & Ancill, 1991; Cooper, 1993; Gerdner, & Buckwalter, 1994; Lai, 1999; Sloane et al.,1997; White, Merrie, & Richie, 1996;). Although a small number of studies were conducted in an adult day care or community setting (Burgeois et al., 1997; Cohen-Mansfield, 1998), the majority of research studies continued to address vocally disruptive behaviour in the geriatric nursing home resident.

Research in the 1990's took a multi-disciplinary approach with a variety of disciplines conducting research into VDB. In addition to the early research that was conducted by nurses, physicians, and psychologists, other disciplines such as social workers, occupational therapists, speech language pathologists and pharmacists began to examine different aspects of assessment and management of vocally disruptive behaviour (Casby, & Holm, 1994; Cooper, 1993; Sloane et al., 1997; Toseland et al., 1997).

Research into vocally disruptive behaviour has continued to grow and expand rapidly throughout the 1990's. Currently there are a variety of approaches, definitions and methods for assessment, measurement and evaluation of interventions for VDB utilized in the literature. The challenge for clinicians and researchers in the new millennium will be to refine definitions and measurement methods and progress to the implementation and evaluation of effective interventions.

In summary, the study of vocally disruptive behaviour from the mid 1980s until present day has proposed various theoretical perspectives and has described the prevalence of VDB in institutional settings, defined VDB, developed a profile of the resident with VDB, and attempted to develop assessment mechanisms and management strategies. A review and discussion of each area follows.

Theoretical Perspectives

In her 1999 article on current knowledge related to vocally disruptive behaviour, Lai points out that although etiologies for the occurrence of VDB have not been identified, various theories have been developed. Cohen-Mansfield and Werner (1997) identified four theories that can be grouped under two main categories. The first two theories originate from the biomedical model and look at diagnosis and disease process while the other two theories are modeled after psychosocial theories and focus on the environment and interaction with others (Lai, 1999).

Biomedical Theories (Diagnosis/ Disease Process)

The first biomedical theory postulates that vocally disruptive behaviour is a result of neurological damages associated with Alzheimer's disease and other dementias (Cohen-Mansfield et al., 1997). Lai (1999) further clarifies that personality changes are believed to be common in dementing disorders and that depending on the area of the brain that is affected a loss of inhibition is produced that activates screaming. Much of the research that was completed in the early 1990's provided evidence of a strong correlation between cognitive impairment due to a dementing illness and vocally disruptive behaviour (Burgio et al., 1994; Cariaga et al., 1991; Cohen-Mansfield et al., 1990; Hallberg et al. 1990).

The second biomedical theory postulates that vocally disruptive behaviour is an expression of physical discomfort or mental suffering (Cohen-Mansfield et al., 1997). Pain in this context is most frequently considered to be physical pain, although some researchers also associate mental pain, for example depression (Lai, 1999). Although this theory has received a good deal of support limited amounts of empirical evidence exist. In 1990, in their pioneering research, Cohen-Mansfield and colleagues identified depressed affect as one of the profile characteristics of the vocally disruptive resident (Cohen-Mansfield et al., 1990). In a letter to the editor, Carlyle, Killick, and Ancill (1991), site three cases where ECT was effective in the treatment of vocally disruptive behaviour in three residents, only one of whom had a previous diagnosis of depression.

Cariaga and colleagues noted in their 1991 study that subjects in the comparison group were significantly more likely to receive acetaminophen, pointing out that pain in vocally disruptive, demented residents may go untreated or under treated and may potentially contribute to the VDB. Cohen-Mansfield and associates in their

1997 study of the typology of vocally disruptive behaviour identify three categories of VDB. Typology of vocalizations was determined for 45 vocally disruptive residents over a 40 day observation period by examining the type of sound (for quality, content and timing), purpose of sound (whether the behaviour expressed a specific need), response to the environment and level of disruptiveness. The first category of VDB identified by the researchers included verbal behaviours associated with specific requests or specific needs, or behaviours associated with pain (such as loud talk) (Cohen-Mansfield et al., 1997).

Further in depth study is required into biomedical theories of vocally disruptive behaviour in nursing home residents with dementia. Potential contributing factors such as physical and mental pain have serious but positive treatment and intervention implications.

Psychosocial Theories (The Environment/ Interaction with Others)   OPERANT LEARNING

The first psychosocial theory that has been postulated to explain vocally disruptive behaviours is based on operant learning. Vocally disruptive behaviour is sometimes seen as operant, whereby the behaviour is reinforced by attention from staff and other residents (Lai, 1999). Several studies suggest that within the vacuum of a nursing home environment that any attention can be a positive reinforcement and that generally vocally disruptive behaviour is reinforced by the way staff interact with patients exhibiting the behaviour (Hallberg et al., 1990; Hallberg & Norberg., 1990; Hallberg et al., 1993).

The second psychosocial theory that has been postulated originates from the findings of various researchers and to date have received the most research attention in the 1990's. This theory is related directly to the nursing home environment and postulates that vocally disruptive behaviour is an outcome of sensory deprivation and social isolation (Lai, 1999). This theory has been researched over the last 10 years in a number of studies conducted in Sweden by Hallberg and associates. Their work

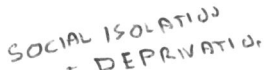

SOCIAL ISOLATION + DEPRIVATION

examines sensory deprivation and social isolation in terms of the nursing home environment and staff approaches and interactions with vocally disruptive residents (Hallberg et al., 1990; Hallberg & Norberg, 1990; Hallberg et al., 1993; Hallberg, Edberg, Nordmark et al, 1993; Holst et al., 1997). In their 1990 study Hallberg and colleagues reported that other than hands on care, 71% of the resident's time was spent alone or in inactivity (Hallberg et al., 1990). They postulate that demented persons suffer from sensory deprivation as a result of their inability to interact with the environment, both in the physical sense and in the social sense (Lai, 1999). Hallberg and associates research supports that the decreased ability to process sensory input as a consequence of aging and disease process, and monotonous institutional life evoke feelings of fear, boredom and loneliness that subsequently result in the manifestation of vocally disruptive behaviour to express negative emotions and stimulate self (Hallberg et al., 1990; Hallberg & Norberg, 1990; Hallberg et al., 1993; Hallberg, Edberg, Nordmark et al., 1993; Holst et al., 1997; Lai, 1999).

SELF-STIMULATION

Cohen-Mansfield and Werner (1997) found that social isolation produced a specific typology of vocally disruptive behaviour that was associated with self-stimulation such as loud singing and tended to be manifested on a constant basis. Sloane and colleagues (1997) go one step further and postulate that VDB can either be a product of environmental under-stimulation/isolation or that it can also be a result of environmental over-stimulation. Over-stimulation can occur during care, group activities and in the late afternoon at change of shift (Sloane et al., 1997).

Related research examined potential environmental influences in terms of care giving activities, staff approaches and lack of social stimulation in the nursing home environment. Research topics have included staff approach during hands on care, time spent providing hands on care, time spent socially interacting, staff attitudes and feelings, effect of staff training programs on reducing VDB and identification of commonly used interventions (Cohen-Mansfield et al. 1990; Hallberg et al., 1990; Hallberg et al., 1993; Wallace, 1994; Rantz, 1994; Whall et al., 1992).

Definitions of Vocally Disruptive Behaviours

Early case studies attempted to define vocally disruptive behaviour utilizing a variety of descriptive terms. These included terms such as screaming and shouting, calling out and loud, repetitive verbal utterances (Christie & Ferguson, 1988; Stokes, 1988; Zachow, 1984;).

In 1988, Canadian researchers, Ryan and associates conducted a study in a long term care facility that was aimed specifically at examining the prevalence and describing the characteristics of vocally disruptive behaviour. The definition developed during this project has been used frequently in research studies that followed in the late 1980's and 1990's. The person exhibiting VDB was described as; "The noisy patient shows a chronic pattern of perseverative verbal behaviour. The pattern may be continuous or intermittent, goal directed or without apparent purpose. It may vary in loudness, content and impact" (Ryan et al, 1988, pp.380). In addition, they identified six categories of noise making: "1) noise making which appears purposeless and perseverative, 2) noise making which is a response to the environment, 3) noise making which appears directed toward eliciting a response from the environment, 4) chatterbox noise making in the context of deafness and 6) other noise making" (Ryan et al,1988, pp. 380).

Between 1986 and 1988, Cohen-Mansfield and colleagues grouped behavioural disturbances into 3 categories based upon their characteristics, one of which defined vocally disruptive behaviour; "a) physically aggressive behaviours; b) physically non-aggressive behaviours; and c) verbally agitated behaviours"(Cohen-Mansfield et al, 1992, pp. 223-224). They described verbally agitated behaviours as "complaining, constant requests for attention, negativism, repetitious sentences or questions and screaming" (Cohen-Mansfield et al pp. 224). Cariaga and colleagues (1991) developed a definition of vocally disruptive behaviour during the course of their research that described VDB as "persistent moans and groans, screams, abusive language (profanities), repetitive verbalizations and negativism" (Cariaga et al., 1991, pp.502).

Many of the studies conducted between 1990 and 1997 quote one or more of the above definitions for vocally disruptive behaviour, while many other studies do not provide a specific definition and simply state that staff were asked to identify patients or residents who were vocally disruptive.

In the latter part of the 1990's, Sloane and colleagues add a further dimension to the construct of vocally disruptive behaviour by differentiating between verbal agitation and verbal aggression. Verbal agitation is described as complaining, screaming, yelling, constant requests for attention and repetitious noises, words or phrases. Verbal aggression is defined differently as hostile and accusatory in nature and often threatens harm (usually time limited and in response to a perceived threat) (Sloane et al., 1997).

A number of questions can be posed when reviewing the various definitions used to describe vocally disruptive behaviour. Do they define the same construct? Is vocally disruptive behaviour a single construct? Cohen-Mansfield and Werner (1997) state that their research into the typology of vocally disruptive behaviour demonstrates that VDB is not a single construct. They identify three main groups of vocally disruptive behaviour with different etiologies; "1) verbal behaviours associated with specific requests or specific needs, including behaviours associated with the performance of ADLs (such as chatting); or behaviours associated with pain, the need to be fed or put in bed (such as loud talk); 2) verbal behaviours not associated with specific requests but with general, undefined needs, including calling for attention (such as inappropriate verbal) or hallucinations (such as mumbling and disruptive talk); 3) verbal behaviours associated with self-stimulation, such as loud singing" (Cohen-Mansfield et al., 1997, pp.1086). They also point out that clinical staff members willing to manage these VDB have to consider the etiological reasons associated with each one and treat them as separate behaviours requiring different interventions.

Lai (1999), points out that it is difficult to compare results of many of the studies to date due to the fact that each has used a different operational definition of vocally disruptive behaviour. More research is required to clearly define the constructs of VDB so that studies conducted in the future are comparable and generalizable.

Prevalence of Vocally Disruptive Behaviours

Early studies, prior to 1988, either did not report on the prevalence of vocally disruptive behaviour or provided only simple estimates of the prevalence of VDB. Ryan and colleagues (1988) provided, in addition to a definition of vocally disruptive behaviour, a systematic report on the prevalence of vocally disruptive behaviour based on research. Their study which included a pilot and a replication study was conducted in a large Canadian long term care facility. They reported a prevalence rate of 29 % (117 out of 400 residents) in the pilot study and 31% (196 out of 600 residents) in the replication study (Ryan et al., 1988).

A number of studies that followed in the 1990's also reported on the prevalence of vocally disruptive behaviour in an institutional setting. Cohen-Mansfield, Werner, and Marx (1990) reported in their survey of 408 residents from a long term care facility in the United States that 25% of the residents screamed at least four times per week. Results of their research indicated that 15% of the 408 residents (n = 62) were classified as high-frequency screamers; these residents screamed at a frequency of at least once or twice a day (Cohen-Mansfield et al,1990). Another 10% of the 408 residents (n = 39) were rated as screaming four or five times per week (Cohen-Mansfield et al,1990). Cariaga and colleagues (1988, 1991) reported a much lower prevalence rate of 11% in a sample of 350 residents in two county nursing homes, also in the United States.

These three landmark studies have reported that 11%-31% of residents display VDB. These numbers are widely accepted and are quoted consistently in other research studies. Since 1990, research specifically focused on prevalence of vocally disruptive behaviour has been limited. As Lai (1999) points out, however, true prevalence of vocally disruptive behaviour is difficult to ascertain due to several factors.

The varying definitions used in research studies to date suggest that one should use caution in interpreting reported prevalence. Another important note is that the majority of research examining prevalence of vocally disruptive behaviour was conducted in a personal care home, psychogeriatric or special needs setting. Prevalence, therefore, should not be generalized between or beyond these settings. Further research into the true prevalence of vocally disruptive behaviour is required using a consistent operational definition. In addition, studies have yet to be conducted that will examine the prevalence in adult day care and community settings.

Profile of the Vocally Disruptive Resident

Cohen-Mansfield, Werner and Marx (1990) conducted pioneering research to yield an overall picture of the vocally disruptive resident. Results of this early research found that screaming was positively and significantly related to depressed affect, cognitive impairment, activities of daily living (ADL) impairment, total number of falls, sleep problems, and perceived levels of pain (Cohen-Mansfield et al., 1990). In this same study, Cohen-Mansfield and colleagues found that residents with certain characteristics tended to scream more than others. These characteristics included incontinence, past experience of a life threatening event, and a poor quality of social network (Cohen-Mansfield et al.). They also found that there was no significant relationship between gender and VDB and between marital status and VDB (Cohen-Mansfield et al.). Subsequent research has provided support for some but not all of the profile characteristics identified by Cohen-Mansfield and colleagues in this early study. In addition, research studies that followed in the 1990's have identified other personal and environmental characteristics that create a profile of the vocally disruptive resident.

Cohen-Mansfield and colleagues found that a significant degree of cognitive impairment (due to dementia) was positively correlated with the profile of the vocally disruptive resident. This finding has been supported consistently throughout the literature. Studies continue to find that a significant degree of cognitive impairment (due to dementia) is positively correlated with vocally disruptive behaviour (Beck et a., 1998; Burgio, 1997; Burgio et al., 1994; Cariaga et al., 1991; Hallberg et al., 1990; Sloane et al., 1997; Sloane et al., 1999). Despite the fact that variation is seen in the operational definitions of vocally disruptive behaviour used in different research studies, the link between cognitive impairment due to dementia and vocally disruptive behaviour appears to be strong and has been consistently well supported.

The majority of the studies used the Mini Mental State Exam (MMSE) to assess degree of cognitive impairment due to dementia (Burgio, 1997; Burgio et al., 1994; Cariaga et al., 1991), while others used a variety of methods including the Organic Brain Scale (OBS) (Hallberg et al.,1990), the Brief Cognitive Rating Scale (BCRS) (Cohen-Mansfield et al., 1990), and diagnosis of dementia from the medical record (Sloane et al., 1999). Although different methods of determining the presence of cognitive impairment due to dementia have been utilized, results of the research studies appear to consistently support the association.

The second profile characteristic of the vocally disruptive resident that has received consistent support in the literature is the presence of functional impairment and the need to receive assistance with activities of daily living (ADLs). Cohen-Mansfield and colleagues (1990) assessed the ability to perform six activities of daily living; bathing, eating, toileting, grooming, dressing and walking and found that screaming was significantly and positively related to ADL impairment (Cohen-Mansfield et al., 1990). Hallberg and colleagues (1990) conducted a study in Sweden to specifically examine and describe the functional impairment of vocally disruptive patients compared with controls as well as to examine the clusters or patterns of functional impairment in vocally disruptive residents compared with controls. The most important finding in their study supported those of Cohen-Mansfield. Their study found that vocally disruptive behaviour was related to a high degree of physical dependence and need for assistance with bathing, dressing, toileting, feeding, and mobility (Hallberg et al., 1990). Cariaga and colleagues' 1991 study provided further support to suggest that residents in nursing homes who display disruptive vocalizations require assistance in three or more activities of daily living such as feeding, dressing, hygiene, bathing, mobility and toileting (Cariaga et al., 1991).

These two main profile characteristics of the vocally disruptive resident, that of being cognitively impaired (due to dementia) and functionally dependent, have become widely accepted by researchers studying VDB. Following these three landmark studies, the majority of research that was conducted between 1992 and 1999 accepted these associations with cognitive status and functional status and began to examine other profile characteristics or aspects of vocally disruptive behaviours. In 1999, Sloane and colleagues conducted a research study that provided further support for the correlation between VDB, cognitive impairment and functional dependence when they found that subjects who were identified as severe disruptive vocalizers tended to have dementia and to be dependent in most activities of daily living (Sloane et al, 1999).

In the same study, Sloane and colleagues found that the most severe disruptive vocalizers had multiple medical problems, were more likely to be physically restrained and were being given psychotropic medications (Sloane et al., 1999). These results have been supported to lesser and varying degrees and still require further research. One study conducted by Cohen-Mansfield and colleagues also found a correlation to multiple medical diagnosis (Cohen-Mansfield et al., 1992).

Use of physical restraints and the link to VDB has not been studied in depth to date, although two studies have found physical restraints were in use with a high percentage of the vocally disruptive residents (Burgio et al., 1994; Kolanowski, Garr, Evans & Strumpf, 1998). These studies do not report the reason that restraints were applied and whether the vocally disruptive behaviour occurred as a result of the restraints. Two studies support the correlation between the use of psychotropic medications and increased vocally disruptive behaviour (Burgio et al., 1996; Cariaga et al., 1991), while another study reported that the use of psychotropic drugs during a 14 day period of observation was not significantly higher (Hallberg et al., 1990).

The profile characteristic of sleep disturbances in the vocally disruptive resident as suggested by Cohen-Mansfield and colleagues in 1990, also received some support in other early studies (Cariaga et al., 1991; Hallberg et al., 1990). Hallberg and associates reported a correlation between the presence of vocally disruptive behaviour and the presence of nocturnal fluctuations. Results of the study conducted by Cariaga and associates show that vocally disruptive residents were more likely to experience a sleep disturbance such as difficulty falling asleep, awakening frequently during the night or confusing days and nights.

Gender has not yet been determined as a profile characteristic for VDB. Cohen-Mansfield and colleagues' 1990 study along with two other studies report no support for gender as a profile characteristic for vocally disruptive residents (Cariaga et al., 1991; Hallberg et al. 1990). However, two later research studies, one by Cohen-Mansfield and associates (1992) and one by Burgio (1997) reported that vocally disruptive residents tended to be female.

Two potentially significant profile characteristics that have not yet received notable research attention are depression and pain, both of which have serious treatment and intervention implications if found to be associated with vocally disruptive behaviour. Pain as a potential cause or contributing factor to vocally disruptive behaviour is discussed in fewer studies. Cariaga and colleagues (1991) noted as a part of their study examining prevalence and profile characteristics that subjects in the comparison group were significantly more likely to receive acetaminophen, raising the question of untreated or under treated pain possibly contributing to vocally disruptive behaviour. Cohen-Mansfield and colleagues (1997) identified physical pain as one of three main types of vocally disruptive behaviours.

Three other profile characteristics reported in the 1990 study by Cohen-Mansfield and colleagues have also received limited research attention over the last 10 years.

These include number of falls (although decreased mobility is noted in a number of other studies as a functional characteristic), exposure to a life threatening event and poor quality social network (although social isolation has received significant attention and support).

Only one study conducted since 1990 introduced the possibility of additional profile characteristics of the vocally disruptive resident. This research study, conducted by Holst and colleagues examined the link between vocally disruptive residents and previous personality traits. In a small study (n=21), they interviewed families of vocally disruptive residents and found that, as remembered retrospectively by a close family member, a previous personality described as introverted, rigid, and with a tendency to control emotions, may correlate to current vocally disruptive behaviour (Holst et al., 1997).

Assessment and Management Interventions
Assessment

Assessment of vocally disruptive behaviour and development of an effective intervention plan has been recognized as extremely challenging for health care professionals. Early literature provided readers with case study examples of assessment and intervention strategies that were successful for one individual (Christie & Ferguson, 1988; Zachow, 1984).

Pioneering studies from 1988-1991 began to lay the groundwork for assessment of VDB by attempting to define the behaviour and identify profile characteristics of the vocally disruptive resident (Cariaga et al., 1991; Cohen-Mansfield et al., 1990; Hallberg et al. 1990; Ryan et al., 1988). Over the next 6-7 years assessment both clinically and in research studies consisted of identifying that vocally disruptive behaviour was occurring according to one of the definitions/ classification systems developed from early research. Clinicians and researchers would base their assessment and development of intervention strategies on the general theory (biomedical or psychosocial) they were most familiar with or felt to be appropriate to the situation. Assessment tools such as agitation and aggression inventories and behaviour graphs were available and frequently utilized by health care professionals. There was no tool available to specifically assess vocally disruptive behaviour.

In the early 1990's, little research focused on assessment of the typology of the vocally disruptive behaviour. In 1991 Cariaga and colleagues did identify that different types of vocally disruptive behaviour do exist. Two years later, in 1993, Hallberg and associates attempted to provide a thorough description of vocally disruptive behaviours in terms of amount, duration, level, content and type by analyzing continuous tape recordings of daytime vocal activity in institutionalized, severely demented, vocally disruptive patients. However, it was not until 1997 that researchers began to closely examine the need to develop a more comprehensive approach to assessment. Researchers and clinicians began to recognize that, in order to determine the most likely cause/contributing factors and therefore the most appropriate intervention strategies, more than just identifying that VDB is occurring was required. A comprehensive assessment of VDB would need to include determination of the specific typology of the vocally disruptive behaviour.

Cohen-Mansfield and Werner (1997) demonstrated in their study examining the typology of vocally disruptive behaviour that VDB is not a single construct. Results of their research led them to conclude that clinical staff members willing to manage these VDB have to consider the etiological reasons associated with each one and treat them as separate behaviours requiring different interventions (Cohen-Mansfield et al., 1997). In their study, Cohen-Mansfield and colleagues identified two main groups of vocally disruptive behaviour; those that are verbal (inappropriate loud talk, loud singing, loud cursing, disruptive talk, chatting, mumbling and yelling) and those that are non-verbal (groaning, moaning, howling and sighing). Non verbal vocally disruptive behaviour was most often associated with advanced cognitive impairment due to dementia and it was found to be difficult to attribute any meaning to these behaviours (Cohen-

TWO-TYPOLOGIES

Mansfield et al..). Cohen-Mansfield and associates point out in their research report that as the cognitive ability of the elderly residents deteriorated, their VDB became less verbal and seemed less related to specific needs or purposes. Within the group of vocally disruptive behaviour considered verbal, three main groups can be identified:

"1. Verbal behaviours associated with specific requests or specific needs, including behaviours associated with the performance of ADLs (such as chanting); or behaviours associated with pain, the need to be fed, or put in bed (such as loud talk)

2. Verbal behaviours not associated with specific requests but with general undefined needs, including calling for attention (such as inappropriate verbal) or hallucinations (such as mumbling and disruptive talk).

3. Verbal behaviours associated with self-stimulation, such as loud singing" (Cohen-Mansfield et al., 1997 pp. 1086).

The typology of vocally disruptive behaviour developed by Cohen-Mansfield and Werner also includes assessment of timing of the behaviour. Verbal behaviours which were identified as expressing self-stimulation tended to be manifested on a constant basis, while verbal behaviours which reflected a specific need or purpose tended to display a specific pattern, usually associated with the performance of ADLs or the presence of physical pain (Cohen-Mansfield et al., 1997). Cohen-Mansfield and Werner developed and validated a tool for the assessment of the typology of VDB as well as validated the typology against Ryan and colleagues 1988 classification system.

In another 1997 article, Sloane and colleagues report the results of a consensus meeting convened to provide guidelines for clinicians and recommendations for researchers. Assessment guidelines are provided along with general management principles and specific intervention strategies. Although these guidelines do not focus in the same degree of detail as Cohen-Mansfield and colleagues on the typology of the VDB, they do provide clinical staff with direction and encourages them to pay careful attention to the type of sounds in the disruptive vocalization including loudness, timing, frequency, content, tone. As well, non-verbal cues and the context of the situation is emphasized (Sloane et al., 1997).

Management Interventions

Although not always introduced to manage a specific typology of vocally disruptive behaviour as identified by Cohen-Mansfield and colleagues, researchers from several different disciplines have identified and studied a wide variety of management interventions in relation to vocally disruptive behaviours. The studies that report on management interventions fall into several broad categories; those interventions observed or reported to be used by staff and those interventions applied and examined in research studies.

One of the most controversial management techniques, as with other types of disruptive and agitated behaviour, is the use of medication or chemical restraints. Until the 1990's, residents in personal care home settings who displayed significant VDB were treated with psychotropic drugs. Burgio and colleagues (1996) review research findings that show pharmacology to be only moderately effective. Both Burgio and associates (1996) and Cooper (1993) review recommendations from the Omnibus Budget Reconciliation Act (OBRA) which requires careful documentation and justification of the usage of pharmacological agents in nursing home patients in the USA. These guidelines state specifically that residents displaying a behavioural disturbance must also exhibit psychotic symptoms or be a danger to themselves or others before neuroleptic medication can be prescribed (Burgio et al., 1996). The OBRA guidelines also state that only constant screaming has any justification for the use of medication (Cooper, 1993). These guidelines recommend that, as an alternative to medication, behaviour intervention and staff training be used as the first approach to managing behaviour problems

It has become common practice in most institutions over the last 5-10 years to provide staff who are employed on special needs or psychogeriatric units with specialized training in managing a variety of types of disruptive behaviour. A large number of studies have been conducted that continue to support the need for ongoing specialized training for staff who work with residents with dementia. In support of training staff to manage VDB, Wallace demonstrated with a small number of health care aids that a training program specific to VDB did appear to decrease the behaviour (Wallace, 1994).

In focus groups conducted in 1994, Rantz found staff identified four basic intervention categories they used in managing vocally disruptive and other disruptive behaviour. These included: helping the resident to interpret reality, maintaining normalcy, meeting basic needs and managing behaviour disturbances by identifying and communicating warning signs. Staff did state, however, that they felt tolerating or ignoring inappropriate repetitive speech was an appropriate benevolent intervention.

Sloane and colleagues (1997) provide a reference table of interventions for members of a multi-disciplinary team to follow based on a consensus meeting of clinicians and researchers. The table summarizes recommended intervention strategies according to the trigger of vocalization. Similar to Cohen-Mansfield and colleagues (1997) assessment of typology of the VDB, Sloane and associates (1997) encourage health care professionals to base their interventions on a careful assessment of factors that may be causing the VDB. These individualized interventions are designed to effect the environment around the resident in order to decrease or eliminate the potential causes/contributing factors to the VDB rather than trying to change the individual profile characteristics of the resident.

Some of the most frequently recommended intervention activities have been utilized by clinicians with varying degrees of success. These are well summarized by Cooper and include: a multi-generational approach with full-time daycare centres integrated into nursing homes, pet therapy, plant therapy, art therapy, exercise therapy, attendance at worship services, dance therapy and music therapy (Cooper, 1993, pp.37). Gerdner and Buckwalter (1994) group many of the interventions for managing VDB under reassuring therapies which include but are not limited to such things as music therapy, doll therapy and individual sensory stimulation programs. They also discuss a group of interventions they describe as environmental modification which address interventions to avoid under or over stimulation for the resident.

Few studies have been conducted to date that scientifically and rigorously examine the effectiveness of many of these specific intervention strategies. Casby and Holm (1994), two occupational therapists, conducted a small study with 3 residents to examine the effectiveness of individualized music therapy. Despite a small sample size, their results were encouraging. Carlyle, Killick, and Ancill (1991), also in a small study with 3 residents, attempted to demonstrate the usefulness of ECT as a strategy to treat a depression that may be a cause or contributing factor to the vocally disruptive behaviour. These and other intervention strategies require further study in the future in order to determine successful outcomes.

Overview of Research Studies
Types of Studies

Thirty seven articles were found in the literature specifically relating to vocally disruptive behaviour. Searches were conducted both by computer using AGELINE, CINAHL and MEDLINE as well as a manual search of journals and review of article references. The search was conducted from 1970 until May 2000. The majority of the 37 articles reviewed in relation to vocally disruptive behaviour were written between 1984 and 1999 and can be classified as research studies. Twenty six of the published reports were based on the results of either qualitative or quantitative studies conducted by a variety of health care professionals. Of the 26 studies, the majority conducted (19) were quantitative with approximately 7 qualitative studies ranging from exploratory studies to naturalistic inquiry. The remaining 11 articles consisted of summary articles, editorials and case studies.

Location of Studies

Evolution of research studies into vocally disruptive behaviour occurred in three different countries simultaneously. The landmark study that looked at definition and prevalence of VDB was conducted in Toronto, Canada at Sunnybrook hospital (Ryan et al, 1988). After this major study, few other studies have been published by Canadian researchers specifically addressing vocally disruptive behaviour. Approximately 2 years later, in 1990, major studies were published from both Sweden and the USA that would also later be considered landmark or pioneering studies. The majority of research studies that have been published since 1990 have been conducted in the USA (20 out of 26), while Swedish researchers have published 5 research reports. Names of several researchers from Canada, Sweden and the USA have become synonymous with the study of vocally disruptive behaviour. Their studies are quoted frequently in the literature. These researchers include: Ryan and colleagues from Canada (1988), Hallberg and colleagues from Sweden (1990, 19993, 1997) and Cohen-Mansfield and colleagues (1990, 1992, 1997) as well as Cariaga, Burgio and colleagues (1991, 1994, 1997) from the United States.

Research into vocally disruptive behaviour has been conducted almost exclusively in institutions, where the behaviour was first identified as being problematic. The majority of studies were carried out in long term care facilities and most often on psychogeriatric wards or special needs types of units that specialize in the care of the older adult with dementia. Caution must be taken not to generalize many of the results beyond this type of setting and client group.

Methodologies
Definition of Variables

As discussed in detail earlier in the paper, clinicians and researchers have used a variety of different definitions of vocally disruptive behaviour over the past 10-12 years. The most frequently used definitions were those described by Ryan et al.

(1988), Cohen-Mansfield et al. (1990) and Cariaga et al. (1991). The majority of the studies conducted in Sweden state no specific operational definition for vocally disruptive behaviours and ask staff to identify residents who were regularly noisy for long periods repeating words, sentences or sounds (Hallberg et al., 1990; Hallberg & Norberg,1990; Hallberg et al.,1993). Other studies simply label the behaviour as screaming and shouting, yelling and moaning (Carlyle et al., 1991), or ask staff to identify residents with a history of disruptive vocalizations severe enough to interfere with their functional abilities and the functioning of the facility (Casby & Holm,1994). Health care professionals must be aware to be cautious when comparing and integrating study results, due to the varying operational definitions used (Beck et al., 1998; Burgio, 1997; Lai, 1999).

Two early research studies by Cariaga et al (1991) and Hallberg et al (1993) begin to examine the typology of vocally disruptive behaviour in order to provide more specific operational definitions of each type of VDB. Concentrated study did not again occur until 1997, when Sloane and colleagues began to clarify the definition by differentiating between verbal agitation and verbal aggression in their report of the results of a consensus meeting of clinicians and researchers (Sloane et al., 1997). Cohen-Mansfield and colleagues (1997) conducted an in depth study examining the typology of vocally disruptive behaviour, validating it against Ryan's 1988 classification. This work provides health care professionals with a more detailed and accurate operational definition both for clinical and research purposes. Further research is now needed to examine individual constructs of vocally disruptive behaviour using consistent definitions.

Data Collection and Measurement Tools – Validity and Reliability

A number of issues arise when examining data collection methods as well as measurement tools and instruments. Secondary data are often used in studies to examine diagnosis, cognitive status, functional ability and disruptive behaviour. One of the reasons for the use of secondary data is the lack of well developed, valid and reliable instruments for this relatively new field of study (Lai, 1999).

Many of the early exploratory studies used a variety of qualitative data collection techniques and methods such as structured and semi-structured observation, audiocassette recording and focus groups (Hallberg et al., 1990, Hallberg et al., 1993, Rantz, 1994). There is always some difficulty in using observation methods to understand human interactions in real life. Timing can be a concern. In most observational studies, the researcher selects specific, time limited observation periods. Some researchers argue that rather than observing only certain staff-patient interactions, observations should be conducted at regular intervals throughout the day or for continuous, lengthy periods of time (Burgio, 1997, Lai, 1999). Burgio and colleagues (1996,1997) begin to make a case for the use of computer-assisted observation and hope to address some of the concerns related to observation. The use of audiocassettes made it difficult to make out what activities were occurring during the disruptive vocalization because the context of the situation could not be observed (Hallberg et al., 1993; Lai, 1999).

Quantitative studies have also used a wide variety of data collection methods and instruments. Very little consistency has been demonstrated in the choice of measurement tools. For example, studies have used a variety of different tools to measure the presence of vocally disruptive or vocally agitated behaviour, the presence of cognitive impairment and functional status and/or degree of impairment. The presence of VDB has been measured using the Cohen-Mansfield Agitation Inventory (Cohen-Mansfield, Marx & Rosenthal, 1989); the Pittsburg Agitation Rating Scale (Rosen et al., 1994) and the Ryden Aggression Scale (Ryden, 1988). The presence of cognitive impairment has been measured using the Mini Mental State Exam (Folstein et al., 1975), the Brief Cognitive Rating Scale (Reisberg et al., 1983); the Organic Brain Syndrome Scale (Gustafson, Lindgre & Westling, 1985) and a diagnosis of dementia from the medical record. Finally, functional status and degree of impairment have been measured using the Rapid Disability Rating Scale (Linn, 1982), the Katz ADL index (Katz, 1976) and the Barthel Self Rating Scale (Sherwood et al., 1977). Some, although not all studies report on the validity and reliability of instruments used. Studies that ask staff to rate vocally disruptive residents using a particular tool do report on inter-rater reliability. Health care professionals need to be aware that none of these measurement tools were designed to specifically measure aspects of VDB. Keeping this in mind, the reader must assess each study individually in order to determine if methods of data collection and measurement tools are valid and reliable.

Samples

Subjects and/or participants that comprised the samples for research into VDB lived almost exclusively in institutions, usually long term care facilities. Most Canadian and American researchers examine VDB in the population of all residents in a personal care home setting (Burgio et al., 1994; Burgio et al., 1996; Cariaga et al., 1991; Casby & Holm 1994; Cohen-Mansfield et al., 1990, 1992; Rantz, 1994; Ryan et al., 1988). Populations studied in Sweden were subjects exclusively from psycho geriatric units (Hallberg et al., 1990; Hallberg & Norberg, 1990; Hallberg et a., 1993; Hallberg, Edberg, Nordmark et al., 1993; Holst et al., 1997). These groups of participants differ in culture from North American subjects and potentially in diagnosis and degree of disruptive behaviour.

There is wide variability in the sample sizes used in research studies to date. Early landmark and ongoing studies conducted by certain groups of researchers consistently used large sample sizes of larger than 300 (Ryan et al., 1988; Cohen-Mansfield et al., 1990, 1992, 1997; Cariaga et al.,1991; Hallberg et al., 1990, 1993; Holst et al., 1997). However, these groups of researchers tended to use the same samples repeatedly. When cross-referencing findings, they are referring repeatedly to the same sample (Lai, 1999). Many of the intervention studies were completed on very small samples, often less than ten subjects (Carlyle, Killick, & Ancill, 1991; Casby, &

Holm,1994; Wallace, 1994). Each study must be assessed individually in relation to sample size and subject group.

Comparability and Generalizability of Results

A number of researchers and clinicians suggest caution in interpretation, comparability and generalizability of research results (Beck et al., 1998; Burgio, 1997; Lai, 1999). Keeping in mind some of the limitations discussed, there is still much that can be learned from the research that has been conducted to date.

Most clinicians and researchers will agree that based on research to date there appears to be two major classes of variables that are directly related to vocally disruptive behaviours. Individual resident characteristics such as cognitive impairment and functional dependence have been consistently demonstrated to be profile characteristics of the vocally disruptive resident in a number of different studies. Environmental context appears to be the second group of variables that are related to VDB. Environmental influences such as staff approach and social isolation or over stimulation have also been consistently identified as contributing factors to VDB in a wide variety of the research projects reviewed.

Those researchers who do advise caution want clinicians and researchers to be aware of two important factors when comparing and generalizing results. Although broad generalizations have been made, operational definitions used are not always consistent and therefore results cannot always be compared. In addition, settings and subject samples are very specific populations. Subject groups are not always comparable and at times the sample size does not allow statistically significant data analysis (Beck et al., 1998; Burgio, 1997; Lai, 1999).

Gaps in the Literature

Following a critical review of the literature to date on vocally disruptive behaviour, a number of gaps in the literature can readily be identified. The first gap identified is in relation to testing of the two leading theories related to vocally disruptive behaviour. Although there is evidence that at times, treatable biomedical causes such as pain and depression may play a role in contributing to vocally disruptive behaviour, research and intervention specifically in these areas have been limited to date. Most research studies have noted a potential association with pain or depression while examining a different aspect of VDB.

Research into the psychosocial theory addressing the effects of the environment, most specifically social isolation, under stimulation or over stimulation have received a little more attention. There is still much to be learned, however, about the personal care home environment and the way staff interact with vocally disruptive residents. Early studies suggest that health care professionals have much to do to improve the overall day to day environment of personal care homes.

Staff knowledge and attitudes is a related area that has been touched upon but also requires further study. Studies that have looked at staff perspective comment that staff are often frustrated and that vocally disruptive residents are the most difficult to care for than other residents. They also note that staff often feel that the resident can control the vocally disruptive behaviour. Further study will be required to determine the contributing role of staff approach and attitudes to vocally disruptive behaviour in residents with dementia.

It is also interesting to note that no studies could be found that addressed the perspective of the informal caregiver of the vocally disruptive resident. If we have identified that staff are feeling frustrated and other residents on the unit angry or upset by the behaviours how does the family member who must come to visit on a regular basis feel? Does this family member need support from members of the health care team and if so, are staff able to provide that support? A small number of studies have examined the family perspective of the care of the institutionalized Alzheimer's patient. Maas and colleagues (1991) and Buckwalter et al (1997) found that family member's perceptions of the staff, facility and care provided can impact either positively or negatively on the relationship between staff and family members and ultimately on the care of the resident. Scott (1991) points out that family members are among our most important resources for learning about the resident. Family knowledge level of the disruptive behaviour and it's impact on the family member's relationship with both their older relative who is displaying the behaviour and the staff is another area that has not been studied to date. Mace (1986) found that families need information and choices provided to them by health care professionals. Lack of knowledge and difficult relationships with staff can result in increased family caregiver stress (Buckwalter, Maas, & Reed, 1997). With this wide variety of identified gaps, researchers and clinicians have much work to do in relation to vocally disruptive behaviours from the resident's, the staff's and the family's perspectives.

CHAPTER 4: DESIGN

Design of Practicum

The design of the practicum consisted of four phases. The first phase involved identification of informal caregiver participants by the multi-disciplinary team followed by individual assessment interviews with selected informal caregiver participants by the student. The second phase consisted of individual teaching and support sessions. The third phase comprised an informal caregiver focus group to evaluate the teaching and support program. The fourth and final phase included revision to the teaching and support program based on feedback provided by the informal caregiver participants.

Definitions

Informal Caregiver – include kin and nonkin who provided care to the elder in the home and who continue to provide caregiving activities after institutionalization (Buckwalter et al., 1997).

Vocally Disruptive Behaviour – will be defined as "the noisy patient who shows a chronic pattern of perseverative verbal behaviour. The pattern may be continuous or intermittent, goal directed or without apparent purpose. It may vary in loudness, content and impact" (Ryan et al., 1988, pp.380).

Phase I - Assessment

The goals of the first phase of the practicum were to: 1) assess the level of knowledge held by informal caregivers of vocally disruptive residents living in a long term care setting, and 2) to examine the perceptions held by the informal caregivers related to their vocally disruptive family member. The student met on an individual basis with each participant to conduct an assessment interview based on relevant parts of the Calgary Family Assessment Model (Appendix A). This phase was conducted at a location of the participant's choice, whether it be in their own home or in a private meeting room at the facility. The student recorded the results of the assessment in note format to maintain confidentiality. Each participant was assigned a code to identify quotes and comments discussed in the results.

Phase II – Implementation of Interventions

The goal of the second phase of the practicum was to prepare and provide an educational and support program that included verbal and written strategies for family caregivers based on the results of their individual assessment. After initial assessment interviews had been completed with all participants, the student developed interventions based on the Calgary Family Intervention Model (Appendix B) including both education and support components. This included an examination of both individual and group needs in order to determine the most appropriate format to deliver education and support. The individual teaching and support sessions as well as the written package of information for participants was based on the results of the initial assessment interviews, guided by the Calgary Family Assessment Model and supported by the literature.

Once the teaching and support sessions and packages were completely developed, the student contacted each participant by phone to confirm their continuation in the project. If they wished to continue, arrangements were made to complete the teaching and support sessions on an individual basis. The individual sessions were conducted either in the participant's own home or in a private meeting room at the facility, on their request. It was expected that there would be 1-2 one hour sessions for each family.

Phase III - Evaluation

The goal of the third phase of the practicum was to evaluate the teaching and support package with the informal caregivers following completion of the program.

This phase involved participation by the family caregivers in a focus group session with 3-4 other participants to evaluate the overall project as well as the material in the teaching and support package. The participants were contacted by the student to reaffirm their participation and arrange for participation in the focus group. The focus group participants were asked to identify parts of the project, teaching /support sessions and package most useful and least useful as well as the features they would change and leave the same (See Appendix D). During the focus group session the student took notes to record the recommended changes.

Phase IV- Revision and Dissemination

The goals of the final phase of the practicum were to revise the program based on the evaluative feedback provided by the informal caregivers. Following the focus group session the student reviewed the notes taken to identify areas in process or content that the informal caregivers recommended be modified. Changes were then made to the teaching and support package based on the participants' recommendations. The results of the practicum as well as the teaching/support program were presented to the staff at Deer Lodge Centre and will be presented to the staff at Riverview Health Centre following the completion of the practicum.

The Setting

The practicum was conducted at Deer Lodge Centre and Riverview Health Centre, two long term care facilities in Winnipeg, Manitoba. The Deer Lodge Centre is a 434 bed long term care facility that was originally built as a Veterans Hospital. Over the last number of years the Centre has begun to admit the general population to their personal care home wings. The facility has six 36-40 bed personal care units, one of which is considered a Special Care Unit as well as two 27 bed interim personal care units where residents who are no longer able to manage in the community await placement for another permanent personal care home of their choice. Of these approximately 270 personal care beds, 2 units (80 beds) care for Veterans only (all male wards) while the 4 other units are mixed Veterans and general population.

Riverview Health Centre is a 388 bed long term care facility with 228 licensed personal care home beds. Of these 228 beds, there are four general personal care units with 42 residents and 2 Special Care Units with 30 beds each. In addition to the 228 personal care beds, Riverview Health Centre houses a 10 bed Behaviour Management/Treatment Unit. All personal care units at Riverview have both male and female residents.

The Participants

Ten participants were recruited from a convenience sample of informal caregivers of vocally disruptive residents living on personal care or special needs units at the Deer Lodge Centre or Riverview Health Centre as identified by the unit Multi-disciplinary team (MDT). The sample was also considered self selected as they were approached by a member of the team first to determine if they wished to participate in the practicum. This eliminated caregivers who may have been feeling overburdened or suffering from a depression or dementia themselves. Therefore, this group of caregivers is not addressed in the practicum as they may require a different approach to education and support. The student met with each multi-disciplinary team at Riverview Health Centre and the Clinical Nurse Specialist at Deer Lodge Centre to explain and provide written information on the practicum and request assistance in identifying vocally disruptive residents and their family caregivers. Residents who fit the definition of displaying vocally disruptive behaviour were identified on each unit by the multi-disciplinary team. The name of their informal caregiver was then identified from the health care record by one member of the multi-disciplinary team (the Clinical Nurse Specialist or Patient Care Manager) based upon the following inclusion criteria:

1) their family member/ friend was a resident with dementia who displayed vocally disruptive behaviour and who lived on a personal care home/ special needs unit at Deer Lodge Centre or Riverview Health Centre;
2) their family member/ friend had been a resident for at least one month;
3) the informal caregiver visited at minimum once a week; and
4) the informal caregiver was able to speak, understand and write English.

Information Gathering and Evaluation Methods

The Calgary Family Assessment Model (CFAM) was used to guide the initial assessment interview. Relevant parts of the CFAM were applied by the student as discussed earlier to determine the level of knowledge and perceptions held by each family caregiver in relation to their vocally disruptive family member (see Appendix A).

Demographic information was gathered about the resident by a multi-disciplinary team member (CNS or PCM) and included information related to the resident's diagnosis, length of stay and length of time disruptive vocalizations had been occurring (Appendix C). Demographic information was also gathered from the participants and included the family member's gender, relationship to the resident, employment, visiting patterns and factors affecting frequency of visits (Appendix A).

The focus group evaluation session at the end of the practicum project consisted of questions developed by the student based on the literature (Appendix D). These included broad based, open ended questions to gather evaluation information on what informal caregivers found most helpful/useful and least helpful/useful about being involved in the practicum project. In addition, focus group questions gathered information on informal caregivers' recommendations regarding the initial assessment interview, the teaching and support package, and the focus groups including process, content, timing, and location. The student took notes during the session and recorded the changes recommended by consensus of the family caregivers. Based on the feedback provided by the family caregivers, the student modified the content of the teaching and support package.

Ethical Considerations

A presentation to each multi-disciplinary team at Riverview and the CNS at Deer Lodge was conducted by the student. A written information sheet was provided to each team member of the multi-disciplinary teams (Appendix E). The teams identified names of residents who fit the definition of VDB to the CNS or PCM within one week of the meeting. The CNS/PCM determined eligibility based on the eligibility criteria provided by the student. Within two weeks, the CNS/PCM approached the informal caregiver with a written information sheet (Appendix F) to describe the practicum and determine if they wished to have the student contact them to discuss participation in more detail. If informal caregivers agreed to speak with the student, the student telephoned them to explain the four phases of the project in detail, to answer questions, gain verbal consent and arrange for an interview.

Written informed consent (Appendix G) was obtained from all participants by the student at the initial interview. Each participant was provided with an information on participation form (Appendix G) that included the student's phone number and the student practicum advisor's name and phone number. Information in the consent form explained that names and all other information provided by the participants would be kept confidential and would only be seen by the student and the practicum advisor. It was explained that each participant would be assigned a confidential code that would be used to identify quotes or comments made when writing up the results of the interviews. It also explained that the student would take written notes during the initial interviews and focus group. Any written information would be kept locked in a cabinet by the student for seven years and then be destroyed.

Participants were informed that they could withdraw from the project at anytime. The consent form also outlined that the project would not cause harm to them and may have some potential benefits to them by providing increased knowledge and support. They may also have the opportunity to benefit other family caregivers as health care professionals learn from and use the information gathered in the project in the future with other family caregivers.

Participants were reassured by the student that specific individual information given to the student would not be shared directly with the unit staff or facility management and in no way would affect the care that their relative or friend would continue to receive in the institution. Any sharing of information to other health care professionals or families would be in a report format with the information grouped to protect the identity of individual participants.

Participants were informed that the student was requesting demographic information from themselves that would include their gender, their relationship to the vocally disruptive resident, whether they are employed outside the home, how often they visit and factors that influence the frequency of visits. In addition the participants were informed that demographic information was requested by the student from the CNS or PCM about their family member/friend (the vocally disruptive resident). The CNS/PCM provided this to the student based on the resident's health information record and it included diagnosis, length of stay at the facility, length of time disruptive vocalizations have been occurring and type of unit the resident lives on.

CHAPTER 5: THE ASSESSMENT AND INTERVENTION

Demographic Characteristics

Seven informal caregivers from Riverview Health Centre (RHC) and three informal caregivers from Deer Lodge Centre (DLC) agreed to participate in the practicum. One caregiver withdrew from the study upon the death of her family member just prior to the first interview. Participants included 5 men and 6 women. Two of the participants were husbands of the vocally disruptive resident and four were daughters. The remainder of participants comprised sons, nephews, nieces and friends.

One of the caregivers worked full time, one worked part-time and the remaining eight participants were retired. Three of the participants visited once a week, four visited between 2-3 times per week and 3 participants visited their family member more than three times a week (all three visited daily). Males and husbands visited the most often. Females (daughters) all visited 2-3 times per week. Nieces, friends and nephews all visited one time per week.

Demographic characteristics for the vocally disruptive residents were also examined. Five of the residents lived on a general personal care unit and five lived on a special care needs unit. Seven of the ten residents had a primary diagnosis of dementia with five specifically diagnosed as Alzheimer's dementia. The remaining three residents had a different primary diagnosis but had a secondary diagnosis of cognitive impairment. Two residents were diagnosed with depression. Six of the residents had five diagnoses listed, three residents had four diagnoses and one resident had three diagnoses listed by the staff member who completed the form (the CNS or PCM).

The vocally disruptive behaviour was described by staff as: repeating words or phrases (code 1 & 5); swearing (code 2); calling out (code 4,3,7); screaming with care (code 3);

screaming for hours at a time (code 6); crying (code 7); yelling (code 8 & 9); and moaning (code 7 & 10). According to staff, two of the residents displayed more than one type of VDB (code 3 & 7). The length of time the VDB has existed as estimated by the staff member ranged from 3 months to 2 years. The average length of VDB was one year, four months. Six residents had been vocally disruptive in another health care institution prior to admission to the facility, one had been vocally disruptive since the day of admission to the facility and three developed their vocally disruptive behaviour after living at the facility for more than three months. One resident's VDB had increased significantly in the last 3 months following a surgical procedure. Staff also reported that three residents were significantly less vocally disruptive now than 6 months ago.

The first question on the initial interview with participants asked the family to describe the vocally disruptive behaviour in their own words. Families' descriptions of the vocally disruptive behaviour matched the staff's descriptions in seven cases. The length of time the behaviour had been occurring corresponded in 8 cases. In one case the family felt that their behaviour had been happening for less than 6 months when the staff indicated it had occurred prior to that but with less frequency and intensity than at present. Length of stay of the resident at the current facility ranged from 3 months to 4 ½ years. The average length of stay was 2 ½ years.

Frequency of the vocally disruptive behaviour as reported by staff varied significantly with each resident. This question was not completed for one resident. Those who reported that the VDB was a daily occurrence indicated that the behaviour occurred from once to 20 times per day. In describing the behaviour they also reported that the behaviour for some residents was intermittent and most often occurred with any staff intervention while for others it depended on what other activities were happening on the unit at the time. Two residents were vocally disruptive continually throughout the day or night or for hours at a time while another resident was vocally disruptive constantly in the evening between 1700-2000.

Results of the Initial Assessment

Participants were given a choice of location for the initial interview. Eight chose to meet in the facility either before or after a visit with their family member. Two chose to have the initial interview in their own home. Interviews ranged in length from 45 minutes to 90 minutes. The questions in the interview guide (Appendix A) were developed by the student based on relevant sub-sections of the Calgary Family Assessment Model (see Fig 1, p.11). The structural and functional categories in the model were examined. In the **structural** category, two of the sub categories, **internal composition and context**, guided the development of questions in the interview. **Internal structure** questions were related to *family composition, gender, subsystems and boundaries*. **Context** was examined through questions about practice of religion and use of available community supports. The **functional expressive** assessment included questions that examined *communication patterns* with the vocally disruptive family member as well as with other family members who may or may not visit the relative with VDB. *Influences, beliefs and alliances* within the family were also discussed through questions that examined the informal caregivers feelings and beliefs about how much control and influence over the situation was held by the resident and the staff. Past and current roles as well as the role changes that have occurred between the informal caregiver and the vocally disruptive resident were examined.

Questions that examined the **functional expressive** categories of *emotional, verbal and circular communication* included those numbered from 1 to 8 on the initial interview (see Appendix A). Included were questions asking the informal caregiver to describe the behaviour in their own words and to comment on how they feel and react when they visit, how other family members react to the VDB when they visit and how their vocally disruptive relative responds to them. When asked how they feel when they visit their relative/friend, all informal caregivers reported that it was an emotional experience for them to visit their vocally disruptive family member. Four of the participants stated they found it very upsetting to visit. Participants were upset both for their family member and upset that their family member was disruptive to others on the unit.

"I'm upset for him. I don't like to see him like that. I know he is angry and it upsets me" (code 1)

" I find it upsetting when she disrupts the whole unit" (code 4).

Two of the four participants who found it upsetting at first did say they got used to it after a period of time (both of their family members had been disruptive for over 1 year).

Two participants found it disturbing to visit. One participant stated "It is terribly disturbing, there is nothing you can offer her to help" (code 7). One participant found it depressing when he stated "I feel depressed for her and everybody I walk by. My thoughts are, they are here waiting to die" (code 10).

Verbal and circular communication were examined by asking questions related to their approach when they visit, the reaction of their vocally disruptive relative as well as reaction of other family members when they visit. Six of the participants used some type of ritual when they visited their family member or friend. Reasons given for using rituals included distracting the vocally disruptive resident and providing something structured to look forward to when visiting. Three participants would hold or stroke a hand, arm, shoulders or back soothingly while talking in a low calm voice. All three found this to be consistently effective in lessening the VDB. Six participants used some form of distraction activity. These included feeding their family member, going for walks, going to the cafeteria for coffee, leaving the facility to go to the mall or to the park, reading the newspaper or other favorite book or reminiscing over photo albums. Three participants spent time trying to find out from their relative if they were in pain, felt depressed, or had any other needs.

Half of the participants (5) indicated that other family members had similar reactions to themselves over the vocally disruptive behaviour. Two participants stated that other family members were "shocked" while another stated other family members do not visit at all because of the behaviour. In one case there were no other family members or friends involved. In two cases, the family member's VDB caused disagreements between the participants and other family members (their own spouse in both cases). There appeared to be no difference in reactions of either participants or other family members according to the type or frequency of occurrence of the VDB.

Communication with other family members and staff was discussed in further detail specifically in relation to the development of the vocally disruptive behaviour in questions 6 to 8. Informal caregivers indicated that the vocally disruptive behaviour was noticed first at the present facility in five of the situations and at another facility prior to transfer in another four of the situations. When asked who first noticed or identified the VDB, four participants felt they noticed it first and three felt staff noticed it first. One participant felt both they and the staff noticed it at the same time and one could not remember. Six families had had some discussion with staff regarding the VDB while three felt that although they had discussed the care needs of their relative in general with the staff, they had not yet had specific discussions regarding the vocally disruptive behaviour.

Influences and beliefs of informal caregivers were examined in questions 9 to 14. These questions address the caregiver's feelings and beliefs about what contributes to or causes the VDB and how much control their relative and the staff have over the vocally disruptive behaviour. The questions also asked the participants to discuss their perceptions about how they think the VDB makes staff feel and how it influences staff response to their relative. Regarding control over the behaviour, one participant felt their family member could control the behaviour to a degree, four felt they had no control and four did not know or were unsure if their family member had any control over the VDB. In terms of staff control, three participants did feel that staff had some control over the behaviour, four felt they did not have control over the VDB and two were unsure.

When examining potential causes and contributing factors four participants felt their family member was frustrated. One participant stated "I think he feels he has lost control" (code 1), while another remarked "she is frustrated because she cannot communicate" (code 3). One participant felt at times that their family member's needs were not always met consistently and immediately. One participant felt their family member was bored, one felt their family member was in pain, one felt it was fear related to physical care (bathing, changing incontinent products), while another felt it was more like the person's previous personality but now she was unable to control it. Finally one participant did not know the contributing factors. Half of the families (5) felt that staff feelings do influence the care they provide their family member who is vocally disruptive.

The *context of the environment* was examined in questions 20 and 21 looking at availability and use of family and community supports. Six participants had other family supports available in Winnipeg. Two were receiving help from outside agencies such as the Alzheimer's society and an adult day program support group in dealing with the VDB. Five found their religion a source of support.

Functional expressive *family roles* were examined in questions 22 to 25. When asked about changes in their role since their relative was admitted, three participants stated they found that they had a similar role with their family member before and after admission in that they had primarily provided social support such as visiting and had continued to do so after admission. Four participants were happier as they now found it easier knowing that their family member was safe and receiving the care they needed. Their role had changed and now they were able to visit socially instead of assisting with grocery shopping, appointments and household tasks. Two participants found that their role had changed and now they provided less assistance with daily tasks such as personal care (bathing and dressing) and household tasks such as cooking and cleaning. Despite this decrease in day to day responsibilities, they found it harder to adjust to their new role. Both of these participants continue to assist with hands on care in the facility. All participants had three common responses to the question that asked what affected how often they visit. These included their own health, their own personal commitments or appointments and their own plans for vacation or respite. They decreased the frequency of visits or missed usual visits if their own health was poor or they had appointments, or if they had scheduled planned vacation.

Analysis of Initial Interview and Development of Interventions

In order to develop appropriate interventions based on responses to the initial interview questions, answers were also grouped by gender and by relationship (ie. male/female, daughter/mother, husband/wife etc.) in order to examine themes and determine if educational sessions should be provided in groups or on an individual basis. Based on both the individual and grouped information and guided by the companion model to the CFAM, the Calgary Family Intervention Model (CFIM), the student developed interventions. The CFIM outlines three domains in which intervention by the nurse can occur; the cognitive, affective and behavioural domains (see Appendix B). Interventions can be targeted to promote, improve or sustain functioning in any or all three of the domains of family functioning (Wright & Leahy, 1994).

There appeared to be no differences or patterns according to gender or relationship in terms of the three domains participants required or requested intervention. The need for further information and education by all participants is included in the **cognitive domain** and was evidenced by positive responses to the student offering information and opinions during the initial session as well as to the offer of an educational package at a later meeting. Wright and Leahy (1994) believe that the most profound and sustaining change will be in the cognitive domain and occurs when the family receives information or education that changes their perceptions or beliefs. Each informal caregiver defined vocally disruptive behaviour differently depending on the specific type of VDB displayed by their relative. Informal caregiver participants did not know the overall prevalence of VDB and the majority did not realize how many others were experiencing a similar situation. Most informal caregivers had one or two general ideas of possible contributing factors but were unsure of more specific causes and contributing factors and how they may affect their relative. Several caregivers were also unsure as to the resident and staff's ability to control the behaviour. This information was incorporated into the educational package and printed material along with interventions affecting the two remaining domains. All informal caregivers were commended by the student for family and individual strengths during the initial interview.

There was a consistent pattern among all participants in terms of need for interventions in the **affective domain**. Interventions in the affective domain are targeted at emotions that can interfere with family functioning (Wright & Leahy, 1994). The majority of participants indicated that they often felt alone in dealing with the situation and that it was validating to know that their relative was not the only one with VDB. All participants benefited from the student validating and normalizing their feelings related to their relative with VDB during the initial interview. Validation helps to alleviate feelings of isolation and loneliness and helps family members realize their emotions are not only normal but have been experienced by others in similar situations (Wright & Leahy). Several participants were commended for drawing on other family members for support.

In the **behavioural domain**, interventions are directed at assisting families to behave differently in relation to one another (Wright & Leahey). The major focus for interventions in the behavioural domain included encouraging respite and devising rituals. Visiting rituals and a personal respite plan appeared to be related to the length of time the VDB had been occurring. Those participants who had been dealing with a vocally disruptive family member for more than 1 ½ years had developed specific visiting rituals and plans for respite for themselves. These participants had much to offer in discussion with the student when identifying a variety of rituals that appeared to be most effective, developed on a trial and error basis by the participants. They also shared ideas on how they dealt with feelings of guilt when first developing a respite plan. In the two cases where the VDB was the greatest in the last 6 months, the participants had not yet developed specific visiting rituals. Five participants did not have a plan for respite or a vacation for themselves. All five participants were receptive to discussing plans for respite and options for their relatives during their vacation.

Although the majority of the participants had talked to staff specifically about the vocally disruptive behaviour and no pattern could be seen in terms of gender or relationship, participants identified this as a difficult area for them, needing to balance their desire to advocate for the best for their relative without interfering with or alienating the staff. Two of the participants had not specifically discussed the VDB with staff at the present facility because the behaviour was well established and known prior to transfer, but they had discussed the behaviour at length with staff at the other facility prior to transfer.

The information provided by participants in the initial interview revealed that informal caregivers required intervention in all three domains identified in the CFIM. The intervention was developed and provided by the student as an educational package for the caregivers entitled "Understanding Vocally Disruptive Behaviour for Family and Informal Caregivers" (see Appendix H). Although overall educational and support needs were similar for all participants, the student made a decision to provide individual educational session for two reasons. The first is that each informal caregiver's experience was unique in many ways and each participant was at a different level of coping with the behaviour. Wright and Leahey (1994) point out that the uniqueness of each family member must not be overlooked and although interventions must be labeled, the nurse must never take a cookbook approach, treating all family members the same. The student felt each family member would benefit from individualized attention and discussions encouraged by the educational and support package. The second reason was logistical with difficulties presented in arranging group sessions.

The Interventions: Educational Sessions and Follow-up Phone Call

After the development of the educational/support package was completed, participants were contacted again by the student. All ten agreed to participate in the intervention phase of the project. Two meetings were held in the participant's homes on their request while the remaining eight preferred meeting at the facility again prior to or after a visit with their relative. Intervention meetings ranged in length from 60 minutes to ninety minutes.

The Education and Support Package/ Sessions

The education and support package that was developed by the student was set up in a question and answer workbook format in order to allow for discussion and follow-up with each participant (see Appendix H). The student reviewed the information in the teaching/ support package with each informal caregiver, encouraging and allowing time for discussion and questions specifically related to their family member with vocally disruptive behaviour. Discussion points for participants included: potential causes and contributing factors of VDB for their relative; prevalence of VDB in older adults with dementia living in long term care; common feelings, emotional concerns and experiences, coping methods including hands on interventions or rituals to try to help lessen the behaviour in their relative when they visit and the importance of visiting rituals for themselves and their relative; discussions on how to approach staff and finally discussions about feelings of guilt, how to cope with them and the importance of regular respite for themselves. Sessions were individualized by focusing on each participant's lived experience as well as their perceptions of their relative and of the staff.

Informal caregivers were given the option of completing the workbook portion of the package during the education/support session or taking the workbook home to think about and fill out at a later date. Three participants completed the workbook with the student while seven participants chose to complete it at home at a later time.

Follow-Up Telephone Call

Participants were asked at the end of the session if they would prefer to meet with the student again to review the workbook information and have further discussions prior to the evaluation focus groups. All ten participants requested telephone follow-up rather than meeting again due to other commitments and time constraints. During the follow-up conversations, the student reviewed each question in the workbook format including a discussion of potential causes and contributing factors of VDB for their relative, visiting rituals to lessen the behaviour, approaching staff and visiting and respite schedules for themselves. All ten participants stated they felt the teaching/support package and discussions had helped them to understand and clarify the causes and contributing factors to the vocally disruptive behaviour in their relative with dementia. One participant felt depression maybe a contributing factor and had made specific plans to discuss this with the multi-disciplinary team. Another participant did feel depression may be a contributing factor but was still hesitant to discuss this with staff or the team. Following the education/ support session, four of the participants planned to introduce or try a new visiting ritual. New rituals included slowly stroking a hand or arm or back and talking in a calm, soothing voice, bringing in favorite music and portable stereo, asking staff to put on specific TV programs at certain times of day, bringing in photo albums or family videos, going to the mall shopping and using the sensory stimulation room in the facility. Informal caregivers indicated they chose the new rituals both to provide their relative with positive interaction and distraction. It also helped the informal caregiver feel they were doing something positive to try and lessen the VDB.

Three participants were going to try and change (reduce) their visiting schedule to one they felt was more manageable. Caregivers found that this decision did carry some feelings of guilt with it. The student was able to provide support for their decision and offer alternatives such as a hired companion, another family member helping out with visits or a volunteer visitor. All ten participants had a firm plan for respite within the next 3 months following the discussions with the student while only six had plans prior to the sessions.

The Focus Group

Seven of the participants agreed to attend the evaluation focus group while three declined for personal reasons. One of the seven participants was unable to attend due to personal scheduling difficulties and two participants cancelled the day of the session also for personal reasons. The three participants who were unable to attend did agree to provide the student with evaluation feedback in a brief telephone interview. Four participants attended the evaluation focus group (three from RHC and one from DLC). The focus group was held in a conference room at RHC. The session was one hour in length. Questions were asked related to what participants found most and least helpful about the process and what changes they would recommend in the teaching package (see Appendix D). The student tape recorded the session and took notes about the discussions as was previously discussed with participants during the consent process.

Both those participants who provided individual feedback and those in the focus group indicated that overall they felt the process had been very positive. One caregiver stated that education was very important to families because " if the behaviour was expected it would have been easier to understand and cope with it" (code # 10 q. 9). Another stated "it was nice to have my feelings validated and know that my (family member) is not the only one who is vocally disruptive" (code # 8 q. 9). Participants agreed unanimously that there is a need for early contact and intervention with families and informal caregivers by the staff in the facility when the behaviour first develops. Families felt staff also required more education regarding VDB and supported the student in her efforts to develop an educational session specifically for staff in addition to presenting the results of the practicum to them. Those caregivers who attended the focus group stated it was also good to meet other caregivers experiencing the same behaviours with their family member.

No changes were suggested by the participants to the initial interview either in length of the interview or the format of the questions. Participants found it a nice option to be given a choice of where the interview would occur. All caregivers agreed that a staff member or a member of the multi-disciplinary team should initiate the discussion around VDB as soon as the behaviour develops. Several participants commented that the vocally disruptive behaviour appeared to be accepted or ignored by the staff when it first began to develop.

Participants had several suggestions about what they found most and least useful about the teaching/ support package. All caregivers who attended the focus group agreed that the workbook did not need to be in a workbook format. They would have preferred information and discussion points but felt that the workbook questions were not necessary. The student was surprised at this response, as the workbook format appeared to provide the opportunity for the discussion points that participants requested and appeared to benefit from. Participants did agree that it was helpful to be able to keep the information to review again at home or to review with other family members. Although all participants agreed with the overall contents of the package, they suggested deleting the section on approaching a team member since the package was intended for use by staff with a family member. The student supported this suggestion, as the overall goal of the practicum is to have an available teaching package for staff to approach family with in order to provide education and support when the vocally disruptive behaviour first begins to develop. Participants had several other suggestions related to the contents, which have been included in the revised education and support package (Appendix I). Participants agreed that it might be helpful to further define the word dementia in terminology easier to understand by lay persons. One participant suggested adding "repetitive words or phrases" to the definition as this is the behaviour her relative exhibits while another suggested adding " exacerbation of a previous personality trait". Several others suggested adding "fear of hands on care" to the list of potential causes and contributing factors. They had identified a link between staff providing intimate physical care such as bathing and toileting and the VDB with their relative.

Members of the focus group as well as those who gave individual feedback all felt the visiting rituals and respite were important components to keep in the package and stress with families. Additional rituals that caregivers have found helped their relative included going for a car ride, reading letters (real or fabricated) from friends or relatives and going to the mall to window shop. Those participants who had dealt with the VDB the longest had slowly over time developed visiting rituals and learned to take planned respite but had felt much guilt. One caregiver remarked "when I took my first 3 week vacation, I wanted to come home after the first week" (code 6). Caregivers found it supportive when the student gave them permission to take a regular vacation or reduce frequency of visits. They agreed in the focus group that it would be helpful if the facility could provide a list of names of qualified individuals that could be hired to visit when they are away on vacation. The student is not aware if this is possible or if the facilities would be willing, but will mention the request when providing feedback to the facilities.

Other general feedback in the focus group included several messages for staff to help in understanding how the informal caregiver is feeling. On several occasions both in individual and the group session, participants remarked "listen to us, we know them best" (code 5,code 8). Following a period of discussion in the focus group, participants also agreed that they needed to be encouraged and supported in their decision either to continue to assist with feeding, bathing and other care activities to their relative or to not participate in this part of the care. If a caregiver does not wish to participate in this type of care they should not be made to feel guilty. Those who do wish to participate should not have all care left up to them. One participant reported that his relative's dentures were frequently left out until he arrived, no matter what time of day. Several participants stated that they sometimes felt pressured by the unit staff to volunteer for unit social events and help with fund raising activities. Participants wanted to caution staff in their approach and expectations as these caregivers felt this was another source of stress and guilt for them. Throughout the occurrence of the VDB caregivers found the greatest support from those staff members who were willing to discuss the behaviour openly and who would work with them to try to develop approaches to lessen the behaviour. Those same staff also tended to help them to validate and normalize their experience and their feelings related to the vocally disruptive behaviour.

CHAPTER 6: DISCUSSIONS AND CONCLUSIONS
Discussion, Evaluation, Recommendations and Conclusions

Informal caregivers have varying degrees of knowledge related to vocally disruptive behaviour in an older adult with dementia living in a long term care setting and do benefit from planned teaching and support using a variety of educational approaches (discussion, written material, question and answer). Many similar comments were seen as evidence of the perceptions of informal caregivers in the practicum related to causes and contributing factors and amount of control over the behaviour held by the resident and/or staff. The difference in opinion between the student and participants related to the workbook format for the package may have reflected more the student's learning needs than the informal caregiver's needs. Informal caregivers who have dealt with the behaviour over a period of time have developed positive coping mechanisms through use of rituals and planned respite that can assist informal caregivers that are newly experiencing the behaviour in their family member. Informal caregivers that were new to the experience of VDB had developed negative coping mechanisms. They did not always take respite or vacation time for themselves and they often tried to visit more frequently than planned each week because they felt guilty. This negative coping served to increase their feelings of guilt and frustration over the situation. Positive coping mechanisms included those things that assisted the informal caregiver to feel they were doing the best they could for their relative with fewer felling s of guilt. Caregivers did appear to benefit significantly from the education and support program provided to them as evidenced by their individual and group comments and their statements that the staff and family education sessions should be shared with other personal care homes.

It was interesting to note that it was always females/daughters who were approached by staff to assist with other volunteer and fundraising activities on the units. These family members felt increased guilt and stress when asked even if they were able to decline the request. Males in the group had not been approached to assist with other unit activities. Staff need to be aware of this tendency and attempt to support family members rather than contributing to feelings of increased guilt. All participants voiced a need to be recognized by staff for the care that they did continue to provide in the facility. They also wanted to be involved and felt they had something to offer to the assessment and care planning process when the vocally disruptive behaviour developed.

The student found that it was helpful to know the resident and their specific vocally disruptive behaviour when working with the informal caregiver. Knowledge of the resident and their behaviour allowed the student to have individualized discussion that focused on their relative rather than only general discussions about VDB. The staff member who provides the education and support session needs to know both the informal caregiver and the resident well.

Based on the results of the practicum and information provided by the participants in interviews and the focus group, a presentation and educational session has been developed by the student for the staff at Deer Lodge Centre and Riverview Health Centre (Appendix J). This package was derived from the comments and perceptions of the informal caregivers and therefore may not necessarily reflect what staff might expect in an educational session about VDB. Content of the staff package includes information on defining vocally disruptive behaviour, discussions regarding potential causes and contributing factors, a profile of the resident who may become vocally disruptive, a guide to assessment and management interventions and information on including the family in the care planning process while providing education and support. The staff education package was intended to provide the staff with the information they need to know in order to help them understand VDB and begin to assess and manage VDB in their client. It was also developed to encourage staff to provide education and support to families and to include family in the care planning process. The education package for staff also includes an assessment and intervention flowsheet to assist staff in assessment, planning and implementation of interventions. It has been presented to the staff at Deer Lodge and on one unit at Riverview and will be presented to the other staff at Riverview in the near future.

Limitations

The sample of participants in the practicum were a self selected, convenience sample and therefore the approach for education and support developed here may not necessarily meet the needs of all informal caregivers of vocally disruptive residents, especially where the caregiver is feeling burdened or is depressed or dementing themselves. No instruments or measurement tools existed at the time the practicum was developed to address the specific questions of knowledge and perception of vocally disruptive behaviour. Therefore, the student was in a position of having to develop questions for the initial interview based on the conceptual model as a guide.

Future Directions

Informal caregivers have a lot to share with health care professionals in planning and providing care to their relative with dementia who displays vocally disruptive behaviour. At the same time they need to be supported and have their feelings validated and normalized. The nurse is in the ideal position to provide this education and support. In order to do this, gerontological nurses themselves need to be knowledgeable about vocally disruptive behaviours including knowing how to assess the family's knowledge level, perceptions and feelings. Both qualitative and quantitative research is needed with larger sample sizes to further examine informal caregiver's knowledge and perceptions. Valid and reliable tools need to be developed and research is required to determine if the teaching/support package is a valuable intervention for families.

References

Beck, C., Frank, L., Chumbler, N.R., O'Sullivan, P., Vogelpohl, T.S., Rasin, J., Walls, R., & Baldwin, B. (1998). Correlates of disruptive behaviour in severely cognitively impaired nursing home residents. The Gerontologist, 38(2), 189-198.

Beck, C.K., & Sjue, V. M. (1994). Interventions for treating disruptive behaviour in demented elderly people. Nursing Clinics of North America, 29(1), 143-154.

Buckwalter, K.C., Maas, M., & Reed, D. (1997). Assessing family and caregiver outcomes in Alzheimer Disease research. Alzheimer Disease and Associated Disorders, 11(6), 105-116.

Burgener, S.C., Jirovec, M., Murrell, L., & Barton, D. (1992). Caregiver and environmental variables related to difficult behaviours in institutionalized elderly demented persons. Journal of Gerontology, 47(4), 242-249.

Burgio, L.D., Scilley, K., & Hardin, J.M. (1994). Studying disruptive vocalization and contextual factors in the nursing home using computer-assisted real-time observation. Journal of Gerontology, 49(5), 230-239.

Burgio, L.D., Scilley, K., & Hardin, J.M. (1996). Environmental "white noise". An intervention for verbally agitated nursing home residents. Journal of Gerontology, 51B(6), 364-373.

Burgio, L.D. (1997). Behavioural assessment and treatment of disruptive vocalization. Seminars in Clinical Neuropsychiatry,2(2), 123-131.

Cariaga, J., Burgio, L., Flynn, M.A.,& Martin, D. (1991). A controlled study of disruptive vocalizations among geriatric residents in nursing homes. Journal of the American Geriatric Society, 39(5), 501-507.

Carlyle, W., Killick, L., & Ancill, R. (1991). ECT: An effective treatment in the screaming, demented patient. Journal of the American Geriatric Society, 39, 637-639.

Casby, J., & Holm, M. (1994). The effect of music on repetitive disruptive vocalizations of persons with dementia. The American Journal of Occupational Therapy, 48(10), 883-889.

Christie, M. & Ferguson, G. (1988). Can't anyone stop that screaming. The Canadian Nurse, October, 30-32.

Cohen-Mansfield, J. (1986). Agitated behaviours in the elderly: Preliminary results in the cognitively deteriorated. American Geriatric Society, 34, 722-727.

Cohen-Mansfield, J., Werner, P., & Marx, M.S. (1990). Screaming in nursing home residents. The American Geriatrics Society, 38, 785-792.

Cohen-Mansfield, J., Marx, M.S., & Werner, P.(1992). Agitation in elderly persons: An integrative report of findings in a nursing home. International Psychogeriatrics, 4(2), 221-240.

Cohen-Mansfield, J., & Werner, P. (1997). Typology of disruptive vocalizations in older persons suffering from dementia. International Journal of Geriatric Psychiatry, 12, 1079-1091.

Cooper, J.W. (1993). Managing disruptive behavioural symptoms: Today's do's and don'ts. Nursing Homes, January/February, 35-37.

Finkel, S.I., Lyons, J.S., & Anderson, R.L. (1993). A brief agitation rating scale (BARS) for nursing home elderly. American Geriatrics Society, 41, 50-52.

Folstein, M.F., Folstein, S.E., & McHugh, P.R. (1975). Mini-mental state. A practical method for grading cognitive status of patients for the clinician. Journal of Psychiatry, 12, 189.

Gustafson, L., Lindgren, M.,& Westling, B. (1985). The OBS scale. A new rating scale for the evaluation of confessional states and other organic brain syndromes. Paper at the 2nd International Congress on Psychogeriatric medicine, Umea, Sweden, August 1985.

Hallberg, I.R., Norberg, A., & Erikson, S.(1990). A comparison between the care of vocally disruptive patients and that of other residents at psychogeriatric wards. Journal of Advanced Nursing, 15, 410-416.

Hallberg, I.R., Norberg, A., & Erikson, S. (1990). Functional impairment and behavioural disturbances in vocally disruptive patients in psychogeriatric wards compared with controls. International Journal of Geriatric Psychiatry, 5, 53-61.

Hallberg, I.R., Norberg, A. (1990). Staffs' interpretation of the experience of the experience behind vocally disruptive behaviours in severely demented patients and their feelings about it. An explorative study. International Journal of Aging and Human Development, 31(4). 295-305.

Hallberg, I.R., Norberg, A, & Johnsson, K (1993). Verbal interaction during the lunch meal between caregivers and vocally disruptive demented patients. The American Journal of Alzheimer's Care and related Disorders and Research, 8(3), 26-32.

Hallberg, I.R., Edberg, A.K., Nordmark, A., Johnsson,K., & Norberg, A. (1993). Daytime vocal activity in institutionalized severely demented patients identified as vocally disruptive by nurses. International Journal of Geriatric Psychiatry, 8, 155-164.

Holst, G., Hallberg, I.R., & Gustafson, L. (1997). The relationship of vocally disruptive behaviour and previous personality in severely demented, institutionalized patients. Archives of Psychiatric Nursing, 11(3), 147-154.

Katz, S., & Akpom, C.A. (1976). A measure of primary sociobiological functions. International Health Services, 6, 493-507.

Lai, C.K.Y. (1999). Vocally disruptive behaviours in people with cognitive impairment: Current knowledge and future research directions. American Journal of Alzheimer's Disease, 14(3), 172-180.

Lawton, M.P. (1981). Person Environment Fit. In Miller & Cohen (Eds.), Clinical Aspects of Alzheimer's Disease and Senile Dementia (pp.501-519). New York: Raven Press.

Lazarus, & Folkman, S. (Eds.). (1984). Stress, Appraisal and Coping. New York: Springer Publishing Company.

Linn, M.W., Linn, B.S. (1983). The Rapid Disability Rating Scale- 2. Journal of the American Geriatric Society,30, 378.

Maas, M., Buckwalter, K.C., Kelley, L.S., & Stolley, J.M. (1991). Family members' perceptions: How they view care in Alzheimer's patients in a nursing home. <u>The Journal of Long Term Care Administration</u>, Spring, 21-25.

Maas, M., Buckwalter, K.C., & Kelley, L.S. (1991). Family members' perceptions of care of institutionalized patients with Alzheimer's disease. <u>Applied Nursing Research,</u> <u>4</u>(3), 135-140.

McCubbin, M. & McCubbin, C. (1993). The Resiliancy Model. In Danielson, Hamel-Bissell, Winstead Fry (Eds.), <u>Families, Health and Illness: Perspectives on Coping and Intervention.</u> St' Louis: Mosby.

Neuman, B. (1990). <u>The Neuman Systems Model</u>. Norwalk, Conneticut, Appleton and Lange.

Scott, R.S. (1991). Prescription for professionals. What families love and loathe about how we care for Alzheimer's victims. <u>Geriatric Nursing</u>, Sept/Oct, 234-236.

Rantz, M. (1994). Managing behaviours of chronically confused residents. <u>The Journal of Long Term Care Administration, 22</u>(3), 16-19.

Reisberg, B., Schneck, M.K., & Ferris, S.H. (1983). The Brief Cognitive Rating Scale(BCRS): findings in primary degenerative dementia. <u>Psychopharmalogical Bull</u>, 19, 47.

Rosen, J., Burgio, L., Kollar, M., Cain, M., Allison, M., Fogelman, M., Michael, M., & Zubendo, G.S. (1994). The Pittsburg Agitation Scale (PAS): A user friendly instrument for rating demented patients. <u>American Journal of Geriatric Psychiatry</u>, in press.

Rossby, L., Beck, C., & Heacock, P. (1992). Disruptive behaviours of a cognitively impaired nursing home resident. <u>Archives of Psychiatric Nursing,6</u>(2), 98-107.

Ryan, D.P., Tainsh, S.M.M., & Kolodny,V., Lendrum, B.L., & Fisher, R.H. (1988). Noise-making amongst the elderly in long term care. <u>Gerontologist, 28</u>, 369.

Ryden, M.B., (1988). Aggressive behaviour in persons with dementia who live in the community. <u>Alzheimer Disease and Related Disorders, 2</u>, 342-355.

Sloane, P.D., Davidson, S., Buckwalter, K., Lindsey, B.A., Ayers, S., Lenker, V., & Burgio, L. D. (1997). Management of the patient with disruptive vocalization. The Gerontologist, 37(5), 675-682.

Sloane, P.D., Mitchell, M., Priesser, J.S., Phillips, C., Commander, C., & Burker, E. (1998). Environmental correlates of resident agitation in Alzheimer's Disease Special Care Units. Journal of the American Geriatric Society, 46(7), 862-869.

Sloane, P.D., Davidson, S., Knight, N., Tangen, C, & Mitchell, M. (1999). Severe disruptive vocalizers. Journal of the American Geriatrics Society, 47(4), 439-445.

Stokes, G. (1988). Screaming and shouting. Common Problems with the Elderly Confused, Holden, U.P. (Ed.), Telford Road, England: Winslow Press, 3-57.

Teri, L., & Logsdon, R. (1990). Assessment and management of behavioural disturbances in Alzheimer's Disease. Comprehensive Therapy, 16(5), 36-42.

Wallace, M. (1994). The sundown syndrome. Will specialized training of nurse's aides help elders with sundown syndrome. Geriatric Nursing, 15(3), 164-166.

Weinrich, S., Egbert, C., Eleazer, G.P., & Haddock, K.S. (1995). Agitation: Measurement, management and intervention research. Archives of Psychiatric Nursing, 9(5), 251-260.

Whall, A.L., Gillis, G.L.,Yankou, D., Booth, D.E., & Beel-Bates, C.A. (1992). Disruptive behaviour in elderly nursing home residents: A survey of nursing staff. Journal of Gerontological Nursing, 18(10), 13-17.

White, M.K., Merrie, J.K., & Richie, M.F. (1996). Vocally disruptive behaviour. Journal of Gerontological Nursing, 22(11), 23-29.

Wright, L.M., & Leahy, M. (1994). Nurses and Families: A guide to Family Assessment and Intervention. Philadelphia: F.A.Davis Company

Zachow, K.M., (1984). Helen, can you hear me. Journal of Gerontological Nursing, 10(8), 18-22.

Zimmer, J.G., Watson, N.,& Treat, A. (1984). Behavioural problems among patients in skilled nursing facilities. American Journal of Public Health, 74(10), 1118-1121.

APPENDIX A   code_____

The Calgary Family Assessment Model

Thank you for agreeing to participate in the project. As you are aware, your name was given to me by the CNS/PCM because you have a relative/friend who displays vocally disruptive behaviour.

1. Can you describe the behaviour to me in your own words_____

2. How do you feel when you visit and your family member/friend calls out or screams?

3. How do you usually react to the calling out or screaming? _____

4. How do other family members react when they visit and your relative is calling out or screaming? _____

5. How does your relative/ friend react to you when you visit them? _____
_____
_____
_____

6. When was the behaviour first noticed? _____
_____
_____

By whom? _____

7. Have you spoken to the staff about your relatives/friends behaviour? Yes____
No____ Can you tell me a bit about that? _____
_____
_____
_____

8. Have family members disagreed or had arguments over what has been done to manage your relative/friend's behaviour?   Yes_____   No_____ Can you tell me a bit more about that? _____
_____
_____
_____

9. How much control do you think your relative has over the behaviour? _____
_____
_____

Do other family members feel the same or different? _____
_____

Why do you think that is? _____
_____

10. What do you think may cause your family member to call out or scream?
_____
_____

11. How does staff react when your relative calls out or screams? (what do they do?)
_____
_____
_____

12. How much control do you think the staff has over the situation? _____
_____
_____

13. How do you think staff feel about your relative/friend when they call out or scream?
_____
_____
_____

14. Do you believe staff's feelings influence the care they provide your relative/friend
Yes_____ No_____ If yes, in what way? _____
_____
_____

15. Who in the family do you usually go to when you are upset and need to discuss things? _____

16. Are there any conflicts or disagreements among family members at the present in relation to your relative at DLC or RHC? _____

17. Are there any family members that live here in the city?   Yes_____   No_____
If no, where do they live? _____
_____
_____

18. Do you have regular contact with family members? Yes____ No____ If no, is there a reason? _____
_____

19. Are there family members who maintain contact with your relative at DLC or RHC? Yes_____   No_____   For those who do have contact, how often do they visit?
_____

20. Are you presently involved with any agencies or health care professionals to help you understand the changes that have taken place in your relative/friend? Yes_____ No_____ Who or what agencies? _____
What do they help you with? _____

21. Do you practice your religion? Yes____ No____ Do you find this is a source of support in dealing with your relative? Yes____ No____ In what way? _____
_____
_____
_____

22. How did you help your relative/friend before he/she was admitted to DLC or RHC?
_____
_____

23. How has this changed since your relative was admitted to DLC or RHC? _____
_____
_____

24. Has this changed since your relative has displayed VDB? Yes_____ No_____ If so, in what way? _____
_____

25. What would you like your role to be with your relative?_____
_____
_____

Demographic Information gathered from the Family Caregiver:

1) What is the relationship between yourself and your family member/friend who is calling out?
a) Spouse_____   b) Parent/Child_____   c) Other(specify)_____

2) What is your gender?
a) Male_____   b) Female_____

3) Do you work outside the home?   Yes_____   No_____
   If you answered yes, do you work: a) full time_____ b) part-time_____
   If you answered no, are you retired?   Yes_____   No_____

4) How often do you visit your family member/ friend who calls out?
    a) Once a week_____   b) 2-3x/week_____   c) More than 3x per week_____
5) Please list the things that affect how often you visit_____
_____
_____
_____

APPENDIX B

The Calgary Family Intervention Model

Interventions To Influence the Cognitive Domain of Family Functioning

- Commending family and individual strengths
- Offering information and opinions
- Reframing
- Offering education
- Externalizing the problem

Interventions To Influence the Affective Domain of Family Functioning

- Validating/normalizing emotional response
- Storying the illness experience
- Drawing forth family support

Interventions to Influence the Behavioural Domain of Family Functioning

- Encouraging family members to continue to be caregivers
- Encouraging respite
- Devising rituals

APPENDIX C   code_____

Demographic Information gathered by the CNS/PCM from the Health Record:

1) Diagnosis   i_____

                  ii_____

                  iii_____

                  iv_____

                  v_____

2) Date of admission to the facility Month_____ Year_____

3) Briefly describe the type of VDB_____
   _____
   _____

   Frequency (times per day or week) _____

4) Length of time the resident has displayed vocally disruptive behaviours (in years/months) _____

5) Type of unit the resident lives on:

   General personal care unit_____   Special needs unit_____

   Institution (circle)   DLC   RHC

APPENDIX D
Focus Group Questions

Welcome and thank you for agreeing to attend this focus group today. The purpose of our getting together today is to review the practicum project that you have been participating in. We will be discussing what you liked best and least about your interviews, the education and support sessions and the amount of time you spent with the student.

What did you find:

1) The most helpful or useful about the assessment interview (eg. The first time we met)
   Probes: Think about
   - the length of the interview
   - the questions the student asked
   - where the interview was held

2) The least helpful or useful about that interview
   Probes: Think about
   - the length of the interview
   - the questions the student asked
   - where/when the interview was held

What did you find:

2) The most helpful or useful about the teaching and support sessions
   Probes: Think about
   - the written information you were given
   - where/when the sessions were held
   - the discussions that were held
   - how questions were answered

3) The least helpful or useful about the teaching/ support program

   Probes: Think about
   - the written information you were given

- where/when the sessions were held
- the discussions that were held
- how questions were answered

If given the chance, what changes would you suggest be made to the:

a) Interviews;

b) teaching and support sessions

Thank you again for the investment of your time and energy. It has been a pleasure to work with you.

APPENDIX E

INFORMAL CAREGIVERS' KNOWLEDGE AND PERCEPTION OF VOCALLY DISRUPTIVE BEHAVIOURS IN THE OLDER ADULT WITH DEMENTIA LIVING IN A LONG TERM CARE SETTING

Information Sheet for Staff/Multi-disciplinary Teams

Informal caregivers (family members/friends) of vocally disruptive residents with dementia from your facility are being invited to participate in a practicum titled **"Informal caregivers knowledge and perception of vocally disruptive behaviours in an older adult with dementia living in a long term care setting".** It is being conducted by Michelle Todoruk, a student in the Master's program in Nursing at the University of Manitoba.

The definition of vocally disruptive behaviour for the purposes of the project is " the noisy patient who shows a chronic pattern of perseverative verbal behaviour. The pattern may be continuous or intermittent, goal directed or without apparent purpose"

The goal of the practicum project is to determine what teaching and support family caregivers of vocally disruptive residents with dementia need and/or want. A teaching and support package will be developed by the student based on the information provided in interviews by family members. In addition the family members will be asked to help the student to evaluate the teaching and support program

The project will have four phases:
- The first phase will be an individual interview with family members;
- The second phase will be either individual or group education and support sessions held at the facility for family members;
- The third phase will be a focus group with family members to evaluate the teaching/support program; and

- The fourth phase will involve revision of the teaching/support package and presentation to staff in your facility

It is expected that the project will involve a time commitment on the part of the family of 5-6 hours in one- two hour blocks. Family members who are interested in participating should visit regularly at minimum one time per week and be able to speak, understand and read and write English.

If you know a family member who may be interested in participating or finding out more about the project, please let your Clinical Nurse Specialist or Patient Care Manager know within one week. She will contact the family member within two weeks with more information and if they are interested in participating she will give their name and phone number to the student. The student will then contact the family by phone and arrange a meeting to provide more detail about the practicum and their participation in it.

If you have any questions you may contact either the student or her Advisor

Student: Michelle Todoruk **Advisor:** Dr. Pamela Hawranik
(204) 757-4637   University of Manitoba
                              (204) 474-6716

APPENDIX F

INFORMAL CAREGIVERS' KNOWLEDGE AND PERCEPTION OF VOCALLY DISRUPTIVE BEHAVIOURS IN THE OLDER ADULT WITH DEMENTIA LIVING IN A LONG TERM CARE SETTING

Information Sheet for CNS/PCM to read to Informal Caregivers

You are being invited to participate in a project that will be looking at what family caregivers know and how they feel about their relative who calls out or screams at Deer Lodge Centre(DLC) or Riverview Health Centre(RHC). The project is being conducted by Michelle Todoruk, a student in the Master's program in Nursing at the University of Manitoba.

The goal of the project is to find out what teaching and support family members need and/or want. The student will meet with you for an interview, and then will meet with you again several times to talk about the behaviour your relative displays and strategies for dealing with it. At the end the student will meet with you and 2 or 3 other caregivers to evaluate the whole program.

It is expected that:
- the first interview will take 1-2 hours at a location convenient to you.
- the teaching/support sessions will take from 1-3 hours in one hour blocks either in your home or at the facility; and
- the evaluation focus group will take 1 hour.

The student will meet with you no more than 5 times over the next three months.

Participation in the practicum is voluntary. You may withdraw from the project at any time without affecting the services you and your family member receive from DLC or RHC.

If you are interested in participating or would like to get more information on the project, I will submit your name and phone number to the student and have her (Michelle) call you to describe the project in more detail.

Thank you in advance for considering involvement in the project.

For CNS/PCM__ - You may leave the names and phone numbers on the student's answering machine or tell her in person when you see her.

Student: Michelle Todoruk 757-4637

APPENDIX G

INFORMAL CAREGIVERS' KNOWLEDGE AND PERCEPTION OF VOCALLY DISRUPTIVE BEHAVIOURS IN THE OLDER ADULT WITH DEMENTIA LIVING IN A LONG TERM CARE SETTING

Information on Participation Sheet

You have been invited to participate in a project that will be looking at what caregivers know and how they feel about their relative who calls out or screams at Deer Lodge Centre(DLC) or Riverview Health Centre(RHC). The project is being conducted by Michelle Todoruk, a student in the Master's program in Nursing at the University of Manitoba.

The goal of the project is to find out what teaching and support informal caregivers of residents who call out or scream need and/or want. After an interview with you, the student will design a teaching and support program for you and other caregivers. You will also be asked to help the student evaluate the teaching and support program.

You would participate in three parts of the project:
- The first phase will be an interview with you in your own home or at the facility. It will take 1-2 hours.
- The second phase will be individual or group education and support sessions held at DLC or RHC. This will be 1-3 one hour sessions.
- The third phase will be a discussion group with 3 or 4 other family members to evaluate the sessions. This will take one hour.

It would involve meeting with you no more than 5 times in the next three months.

After all three parts are completed the student will present the findings of the project to the staff at DLC and RHC.

Participation in the practicum is voluntary. You may withdraw at any time without affecting the services you and your family member receive from DLC or RHC.

The student will take notes during your interview or discussions. Only the student and her advisor will see any of the information gathered so that your privacy and confidentiality is ensured. The information will be stored in a locked filing cabinet. Any sharing of information with other health care professionals will be done in report format and all information will be grouped to protect individual participants' identities.

Your participation in this practicum will not harm you or your family member in any. It may benefit you by providing you with more information and support regarding the vocally disruptive behaviour displayed by your family member who has dementia. Your participation may potentially benefit other family members in the future.

The student recognizes the importance of and thanks you for your time and participation. If you have any questions you may call the student or her Advisor

---

Student: Michelle Todoruk   **Advisor:** Dr. Pamela Hawranik
(204) 757-4637   University of Manitoba
(204) 474-6716

APPENDIX G: CONSENT FORM AND INFORMATION ON PARTICIPATION

INFORMAL CAREGIVERS' KNOWLEDGE AND PERCEPTION OF VOCALLY DISRUPTIVE BEHAVIOURS IN THE OLDER ADULT WITH DEMENTIA LIVING IN A LONG TERM CARE SETTING

Consent Form

I understand that I am invited to participate in a project that will be looking at what family caregivers know and how they feel about their relative who calls out or screams at Deer Lodge Centre(DLC) or Riverview Health Centre(RHC). The project is being conducted by Michelle Todoruk, a student in the Master's program in Nursing at the University of Manitoba.

The goal of the practicum is to find out what teaching and support family caregivers need and/or want. After an interview with you, the student will design a teaching and support program for you and other family caregivers. You will also be asked to help the student evaluate the teaching and support program.

I am being asked to participate in three parts of the project;

- The first part will be an interview with me in my own home or at the facility. This will take no more than 2 hours.
- The second part will be individual or group education and support sessions held at DLC or RHC. This will take from 1 to 3 one hour sessions.
- The third part will be a discussion group with 3 or 4 other family members to evaluate the sessions. This will take one hour.

It will involve my meeting with the student no more than 5 times over the next three months.

At the end of the project results will be written up based on the group evaluation and presented to the staff at DLC and RHC.

My participation in the practicum is voluntary. I may withdraw at any time without affecting the services you and your family member receive from DLC or RHC.

The student may take notes during my interview or discussions. Only the student and her advisor will see any of the information gathered so that your privacy and confidentiality is ensured. The information will be stored in a locked filing cabinet. Any sharing of information with other health care professionals will be done in report format and all information will be grouped to protect individual participants' identities.

My participation in this practicum will not harm me or my family member/friend in any. It may benefit me by providing me with more information and support regarding the vocally disruptive behaviour displayed by my family member who has dementia. My participation may potentially benefit other family members in the future.

At the end of the project, if I wish, a summary report will be sent to me. My signature below indicates only that I agree to participate in the project.

I agree to participate in this practicum

Your Signature _____ Date _____
Student _____ Date _____

Michelle Todoruk   Dr. Pamela Hawranik
(204) 757-4637   Practicum Advisor
                              Faculty of Nursing
                              (204) 474-6716

I wish to be sent a summary of the results for the project being conducted at DLC and RHC by Michelle Todoruk titled

INFORMAL CAREGIVERS' KNOWLEDGE AND PERCEPTION OF VOCALLY DISRUPTIVE BEHAVIOURS IN THE OLDER ADULT WITH DEMENTIA LIVING IN A LONG TERM CARE SETTING

Name _____

Mailing Address _____

_____

Postal Code _____

APPENDIX H: FAMILY EDUCATION PACKAGE
UNDERSTANDING
VOCALLY DISRUPTIVE BEHAVIOUR

FOR FAMILY AND INFORMAL CAREGIVERS

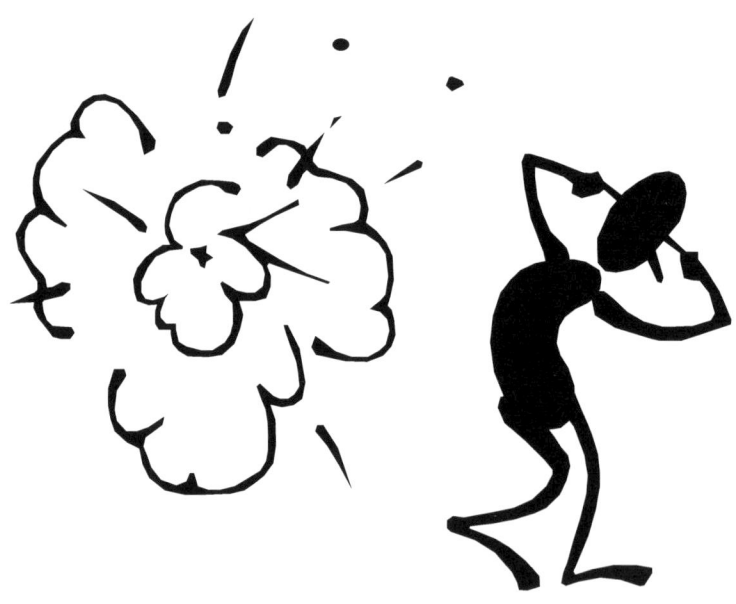

UNDERSTANDING
VOCALLY DISRUPTIVE BEHAVIOUR

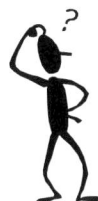 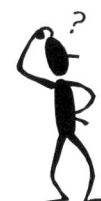 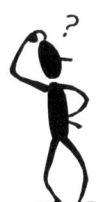

WHAT IS VOCALLY DISRUPTIVE BEHAVIOUR (VDB)?

- Vocally disruptive behaviour (VDB) can be described as:
    - calling out,
    - screaming,
    - yelling,
    - shouting,
    - moaning,
    - crying,
    - or any sounds made by a person that are disruptive to others.

- The VDB may occur once in a while or it may occur almost all of the time.

- The VDB may occur for a specific need or pain, for no apparent reason at all, or for self stimulation.

Vocally disruptive behaviour occurs in 11-31% of residents who have been diagnosed with a dementia who live in a personal care home.

UNDERSTANDING VOCALLY DISRUPTIVE BEHAVIOUR

WHAT CAUSES VOCALLY DISRUPTIVE BEHAVIOUR?

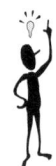 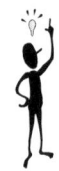 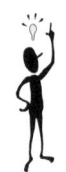 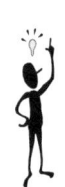 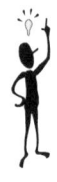

There are several different reasons that VDB may occur. These include:
- Certain areas of the person's brain are affected by diseases like Alzheimer's.
- The person is in pain or is depressed.
- The person is responding to people and events around them (noise, heat, cold, staff and family approach).
- The person's behaviour is reinforced by attention from the staff.

For my family member I feel the contributing cause(s) may be;
_____
_____
_____

HOW MUCH CONTROL DOES MY FAMILY MEMBER HAVE OVER THE VDB?

Persons with dementia are usually not able to control the behaviour. It is an attempt to understand and communicate within their environment. Sometimes your family member may appear aware they are being vocally disruptive and other times they may not be aware of the behaviour. Your family member is not purposely being disruptive.

HOW MUCH CONTROL DO THE STAFF HAVE OVER THE VDB?

Staff most often cannot control the behaviour. They can, however, sometimes contribute to the VDB unknowingly by their actions. Staff are also learning about VDB and what may contribute to it. By working closely with you, the staff can try to determine some of the possible contributing factors for the VDB in your family member. They can then develop a plan of care to follow that will work toward trying to lessen the behaviour.

REMEMBER- Once vocally disruptive behaviour develops, you cannot stop the behaviour completely. The goal of staff and family should be to lessen the behaviour. This may take time and some trial and error. Sometimes it is successful in decreasing the behaviour and other times it may not.

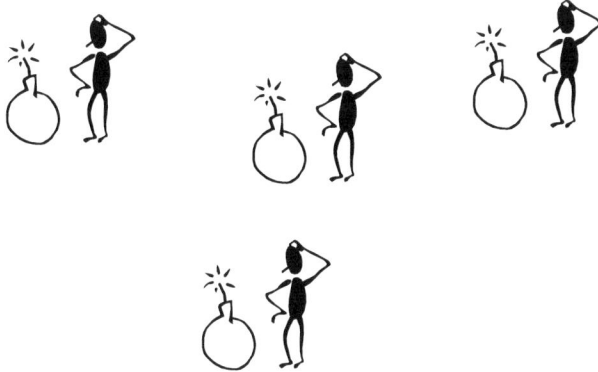

WHAT CAN I DO WHEN I VISIT TO LESSEN THE BEHAVIOUR?

You know your family member best. It is usually a trial and error process.
- Often physical touch and a calm soothing voice or music can help to soothe someone. Holding or stroking a hand, arm, back or shoulders, giving a meaningful hug, singing or humming or playing soft music can sometimes help.
- It is also helpful to have visiting rituals or planned events to help to distract the person and give them meaningful activities in their life. Going for regular walks on the same route inside and out, going to the cafeteria for coffee, going for a walk to the park, reading a special book or looking a photo albums are some examples.

*A visiting ritual I will try (have tried) with my family member on our next visit is*_____

*This did work/ did not work because*_____

HOW DO I APPROACH STAFF TO DISCUSS MY CONCERNS AND HOW CAN I WORK WITH THEM TO TRY TO LESSEN THE BEHAVIOUR?

Decide who you feel most comfortable approaching first. It may be a nurse on the unit who you have developed a good relationship with or it may be the social worker, the unit manager, the physician, the pastoral care worker or any member of the team you feel comfortable with.

Start by letting the person know that you are concerned and would like to discuss the vocally disruptive behaviour your family member is displaying. You may want to request a family conference so that you can discuss your concerns with the whole health care team.

The team member I feel most comfortable approaching is _____

Role play approaching staff to discuss (what I am going to say) _____

I approached _____
I felt _____
I think it worked/ didn't work because _____

WHAT CAN I DO WHEN I AM FEELING UPSET OR FRUSTRATED ABOUT THE VDB?

- Talk to a team member at the centre, the nurse, the social worker, pastoral care or any member of the team you are comfortable with.
- Seek help from agencies outside of the facility (ie. Alzheimer Society, local church etc). It is sometimes helpful to be part of a support group with others who are experiencing the same behaviours with family members. Often friends or the church can be a source of strength and support.

WHAT ELSE CAN I DO TO TAKE CARE OF MYSELF?

- Develop a visiting schedule and do not feel guilty when you are not there or are unable to visit.
- Find time for your own hobbies and activities you enjoy. Do not feel guilty for taking care of yourself.
- Go for walks, read a good book, take a bubble bath, eat well.
- Develop a specific visiting ritual that will give you something to look forward to when you visit.

- Take respite (vacation) time. If you visit everyday, plan to take a whole weekend off every 4-8 weeks. Several times a year plan a period of time (1-2 weeks) away from visiting your family member at the facility. If you are concerned about leaving your family member without a visitor, arrange for someone else to cover, hire a companion to visit or request a volunteer visitor while you are away. A break will refresh and rejuvenate you so you can continue being a caregiver.
- Attend church
- Attend a caregiver support group

My visiting schedule is (or will be) _____
_____

My plan to take care of myself is _____
_____
_____

My plan for respite is _____
_____

I did/ did not follow through with my plan/ Why? _____

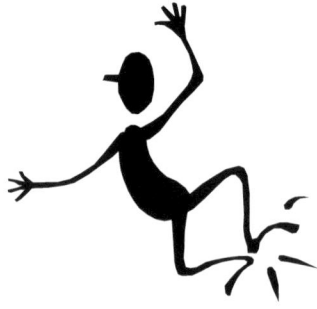

Michelle Todoruk   7574637   April, 2000

APPENDIX I- REVISED EDUCATION PACKAGE
UNDERSTANDING
VOCALLY DISRUPTIVE BEHAVIOUR
FOR FAMILY AND INFORMAL CAREGIVERS

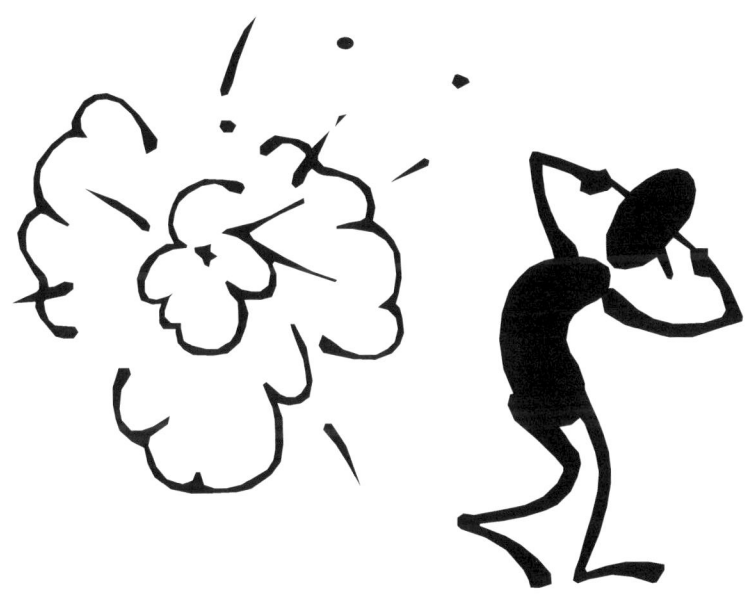

UNDERSTANDING
VOCALLY DISRUPTIVE BEHAVIOUR

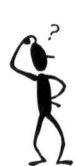 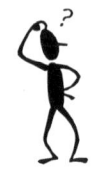 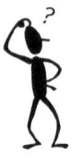

WHAT IS VOCALLY DISRUPTIVE BEHAVIOUR (VDB)?

- Vocally disruptive behaviour (VDB) can be described as:
    - calling out,
    - screaming,
    - yelling,
    - shouting,
    - moaning,
    - crying,
    - repetitive words or phrases
    - or any sounds made by a person that are disruptive to others.

- The VDB may occur once in a while or it may occur almost all of the time.

- The VDB may occur for a specific needs, for no apparent reason at all, or for self stimulation.

Vocally disruptive behaviour occurs in 11-31% of residents who have been diagnosed with a dementia* who live in a personal care home.

*dementia includes diagnosis of cognitive impairment and diseases such as Alzheimer's disease, stroke, Parkinson's disease etc.

UNDERSTANDING
VOCALLY DISRUPTIVE BEHAVIOUR

WHAT CAUSES VOCALLY DISRUPTIVE BEHAVIOUR?

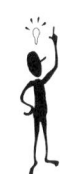 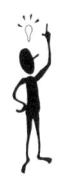 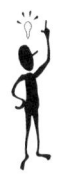 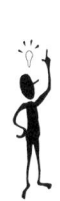 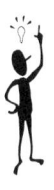

There are several different reasons that VDB may occur.

These include:
- Certain areas of the person's brain are affected by diseases like Alzheimer's.
- The person is in pain or is depressed.
- The person is responding to people and events around them (noise, heat, cold, staff and family approach).
- The person's behaviour is reinforced by attention from the staff.
- It is a previous personality trait that the person can no longer control

HOW MUCH CONTROL DOES MY FAMILY MEMBER HAVE OVER THE VDB?

Persons with dementia are usually not able to control the behaviour. It is an attempt to understand and communicate within their environment. Sometimes your family member may appear aware they are being vocally disruptive and other times they may not be aware of the behaviour. Your family member is not purposely being disruptive.

HOW MUCH CONTROL DO THE STAFF HAVE OVER THE VDB?

Staff most often cannot control the behaviour. They can, however, sometimes contribute to the VDB unknowingly by their actions. Staff are also learning about VDB and what may contribute to it. By working closely with you, the staff can try to determine some of the possible contributing factors for the VDB in your family member. They can then develop a plan of care to follow that will work toward trying to lessen the behaviour.

REMEMBER- Once vocally disruptive behaviour develops, you cannot stop the behaviour completely. The goal of staff and family should be to lessen the behaviour. This may take time and some trial and error. Sometimes it is successful in decreasing the behaviour and other times it may not.

 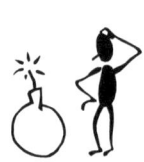 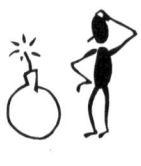

WHAT CAN I DO WHEN I VISIT TO LESSEN THE BEHAVIOUR?

You know your family member best. It is usually a trial and error process.

- Often physical touch and a calm soothing voice or music can help to soothe someone. Holding or stroking a hand, arm, back or shoulders, giving a meaningful hug, singing or humming or playing soft music can sometimes help.

- It is also helpful to have visiting rituals or planned events to help to distract the person and give them meaningful activities in their life. Some examples that others have found helpful are:
    - Going for regular walks on the same route inside and out,
    - Going to the cafeteria for coffee,
    - Going out to the mall,
    - Going for a walk to the park or a car ride,
    - Reading a special book or a letter from another family member,
    - Looking at photo albums,
    - Watching family videos

WHAT CAN I DO WHEN I AM FEELING UPSET OR FRUSTRATED ABOUT THE VDB?

- Talk to a team member at the centre, the nurse, the social worker, pastoral care or any member of the team you are comfortable with.
- Seek help from agencies outside of the facility (ie. Alzheimer Society, local church etc). It is sometimes helpful to be part of a support group with others who are experiencing the same behaviours with family members. Often friends or the church can be a source of strength and support.

WHAT ELSE CAN I DO TO TAKE CARE OF MYSELF?

- Develop a visiting schedule and do not feel guilty when you are not there or are unable to visit.
- Find time for your own hobbies and activities you enjoy. Do not feel guilty for taking care of yourself.
- Go for walks, read a good book, take a bubble bath, eat well.
- Develop a specific visiting ritual that will give you something to look forward to when you visit.
- Take respite (vacation) time. If you visit everyday, plan to take a whole weekend off every 4-8 weeks. Several times a year plan a period of time (1-2 weeks) away from visiting your family member at the facility. If you are concerned about leaving your family member without a visitor, arrange for someone else to cover, hire a companion to visit or request a volunteer visitor while you are away. A break will refresh and rejuvenate you so you can continue being a caregiver.
- Attend church
- Attend a caregiver support group

APPENDIX J

UNDERSTANDING VOCALLY DISRUPTIVE BEHAVIOUR FOR STAFF

Presented by Michelle Todoruk

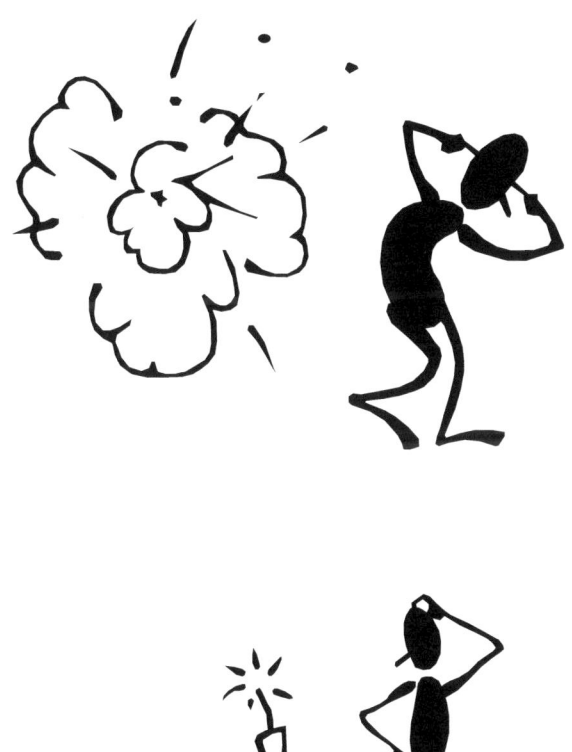

WHAT IS VOCALLY DISRUPTIVE BEHAVIOUR (VDB)?

- ***1960-1980's defined simply as calling out, screaming or shouting.***
- 1988-Canadian Researchers (Ryan et al.) defined VDB as "a **chronic pattern** of perseverative verbal behaviour. It may be **continuous or intermittent, goal directed** or **without apparent purpose**".

VDB occurs in 11-31% of clients in LTC facilities.
Sloane and colleagues (1997) differentiated between;

- **Verbal agitation** (complaining, screaming, yelling, constant requests for attention) and
- **Verbal aggression** (hostile or accusatory and threatens harm)

- **Typology** (Cohen-Mansfield et al 1997) found three main groups with different etiologies
    - **associated with specific needs or pain**
    - **associated with general undefined needs**
    - **associated with self stimulation**

THEORETICAL PERSPECTIVES; *CAUSES AND CONTRIBUTING FACTORS*

Biomedical Theories

- Result of neurological damage associated with dementia

- ***An expression of physical discomfort (pain) or mental suffering (depression)***

Psychosocial Theories

- Operant Learning

(the behaviour is reinforced by attention from staff)
- ***The Environment***
    -Over stimulation
    -Under stimulation

PROFILE OF THE VOCALLY DISRUPTIVE CLIENT

- Cognitively impaired (most often due to progressive dementia)
- **Functionally dependent with ADLs**

Other Characteristics

- Multiple medical problems
- Use of restraints
- Sleep disturbances
- Incontinence
- Depression
- Pain

ASSESSMENT OF THE CLIENT WITH VDB

- **Examine contributing medical diagnosis**
    - Alzheimer's dementia
    - Multi-infarct dementia, CVA
    - Parkinson's dementia
    - Korsakoff's dementia

- Depression
- Psychiatric diagnosis
- Acquired brain injury

- **Rule out treatable medical diagnosis**
  - hypoglycemia
  - UTI
  - pain
  - hypoxia
  - electrolyte imbalance
  - medication reactions
  - delusions or hallucinations

- **Assess the client/ resident for:**
  - communication deficits
  - sensory deficits
  - pain
  - manifestations of sleep deprivation
  - presence of physical restraints

- **Using behaviour monitoring and graphing tools, assess the *typology* of the behaviour in terms of:**
  - amount,
  - duration,
  - level,
  - content and
  - type

- **Using the behaviour monitoring and graphing tools;**
  - look for patterns in the behaviour

- examine the events leading up to the behaviour
- examine the reactions of staff and other clients/residents
- remember to include every aspect of the environment

- **Involve the Family/ Informal Caregiver**
    - Inquire if the person has a past history of poor coping mechanisms
    - Inquire about favorite hobbies, TV shows, music, leisure activities
    - Inquire about things the person disliked or would react negatively to

MANAGEMENT INTERVENTIONS

- *BRAINSTORM* **with every person on the unit who has contact with the vocally disruptive client/ resident**
- **Come to a** *CONSENSUS* **regarding approach and interventions**
- *TARGET* **only one intervention or change at a time**
- *COMMUNICATE* **the plan of care to ensure a** *CONSISTENT* **approach by all staff**
- **Set up time frames to** *EVALUATE* **the interventions**

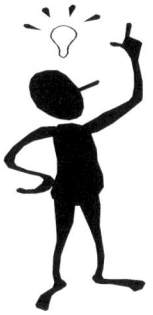

*DO NOT **FOCUS ON HOW TO** STOP **THE VDB, FOCUS ON HOW TO** LESSEN **IT***

COMMUNICATION AND CONSISTENCY ARE THE KEY

CASE SCENARIO

Mr. Y is an 81 year old man who has lived on a personal care unit for 8 months. Staff report he has always been pleasant and co-operative with care. About a month ago, his glasses broke and have not yet been fixed. He has always been an active wanderer, although recently his mobility is deteriorating. He has had several falls recently so staff place him in a geri-chair during the day for safety. Mr. Y started singing to himself in bed at night when he could not sleep. Now he is singing during the day, he seems to be getting louder and staff noticed the singing was often changing to "nurse nurse". Staff moved him to the lounge with the TV on so he would not bother other residents. Just yesterday staff report that he has begun banging on his lapboard.

DISRUPTIVE BEHAVIOUR
ASSESSMENT and INTERVENTION FLOWSHEET

A. EXAMINE CONTRIBUTING DIAGNOSIS

```
_____ Alzheimer's Dementia        _____ Acquired brain injury
_____ Multi-Infarct Dementia      _____ Parkinson's
_____ Korsakoff's        _____ CVA  _____ Acquired Brain Injury
_____ Psychiatric Diagnosis (specify)_____
_____ Other (specify)_____
```

B. RULE OUT TREATABLE CAUSES

```
_____ Hypoglycemia   _____ UTI    _____ Pain   _____ Medication reactions
_____ Hypoxia        _____ Electrolyte imbalance   _____ Depression
_____ Delusions or hallucinations   _____ Other (specify) _____
```

Management Plans/ Date for Re-evaluation _____

C. ASSESS CLIENT/ RESIDENT FOR:

_____Communication deficits (specify) _____

_____Sensory deficits (glasses, hearing aid)_____

_____Manifestations of delirium_____

_____Manifestations of sleep deprivation_____

_____Presence of physical restraints (rationale for use of restraints, length of time on restraints on a daily basis) _____

DISRUPTIVE BEHAVIOUR
ASSESSMENT and INTERVENTION FLOWSHEET
D. ASSESS THE CLIENT USING BEHAVIOUR MONITORING
AND GRAPHING TOOLS

- Using the Behaviour Monitoring and Graphing Tools, graph the behaviour for 3-7 days
- Examine the time of day the behaviour occurs and does not occur _____
- Examine the events (antecedents) leading up to the behaviour to look for possible contributing factors _____

Remember to include every aspect of the environment such as:

-*where* on the unit the behaviour occurs_____,

-*who* is present or nearby_____,

-*what* is staff and others immediate *reaction* to the behaviour_____,
_____,

-*how* does the client/ resident *respond* to staff/others reactions? _____
_____

Determine the frequency of the behaviour and identify patterns in the behaviour_____

Examine the behaviour and whereabouts of the client/resident, staff and others immediately after the behaviour stops

client/resident_____

staff_____

others _____

E. ASSESS THE CLIENT USING BEHAVIOUR MONITORING AND GRAPHING TOOLS

- Using the Behaviour Monitoring and Graphing Tools, graph the behaviour for **3-7 days**
  (**Date started**_____ **Date stopped**_____)

- Briefly describe the behaviour in your own words_____
  _____

- Describe the time of day the behaviour occurs and does **not** occur_____
  _____

- Describe the events (antecedents) leading up to the behaviour to look for possible contributing factors_____
  _____
  _____

  Remember to include every aspect of the environment such as:

  -*where* on the unit the behaviour occurs_____,
  -*who* is present or nearby_____,
  -*what* is staff and others immediate *reaction* to the behaviour_____,
  _____
  -*how* does the client/ resident *respond* to staff/others reactions?_____
  _____

- Determine the frequency of the behaviour and identify patterns in the behaviour_____
  _____
  _____

- Examine the behaviour and whereabouts of the client/resident, staff and others immediately after the behaviour stops **client/resident**_____
  staff_____
  others_____

F. EXAMINE POTENTIAL CAUSES/CONTRIBUTING FACTORS

(check off *all potential* contributing factors)

_____**Depression**

_____**Time** – the person cannot recall a stationary time so may not understand that lunch is in 10 minutes or that it is not time to get up at 3 am.

_____**Timing** – it is better to do intimate care at different times for different people (if someone has always bathed at night do not try to shower them in the morning)

_____**Approach** – staff hurrying, not explaining what they are doing

_____**Word comprehension** – the person may not recognize and understand certain words any longer

_____**Loss of sequence** – loss of sequential thought

_____**Language** – language mix, English as a second language, combining words, reverting to primary language, understanding English but responding in first language

_____**Performance** – apraxia – loss of purposeful muscle movement

_____**Environment** – temperature, noise level, other_____ (circle one)

_____**Disease process**

_____**Race** – the person may not have had contact with persons of other ethnic origins and may be unable to control feelings/comments

_____**Values** – the person may respond better to either a male/female caregivers

_____**Past experience** – the person may have had significant life events occur

_____**Fear of the unknown** - use old memories to decrease stress

_____**Being hurt /having trust for caregivers**

_____**Bombarding** - too much stimuli at once, instructions must be simplistic and given one step at a time

_____**Sundown syndrome** – exhaustion, light source/shadows change

_____**Lifestyle** – the same event can trigger different responses for different people

_____**Old behaviour** – the person may revert to past coping mechanisms

_____**Physical discomfort** – pain, too hot, too cold

_____**Control** - we all need to feel some control over our situation

_____**Busy** – the person may be busy with a past orientation

_____**Progressive agitation** – the person may become more agitated each time staff makes a request of them that they cannot understand/ manage

_____**Confined** – restraint devices, security doors

_____**False cueing**–asking someone to void in bed, on bedpan)or in a chair(commode)

_____**Sensory loss** – decreased hearing, vision, sense of smell

_____**Bored/Increased energy** – under stimulation

_____**Medications** –medications used to decrease agitation may actually increase it.

_____**Personality conflict** – who the person THINKS you are

_____**Pressure** - staff putting pressure on the person by giving tasks that are too complex or hurrying

_____**Mimicking** – if the stimuli is too intense the person cannot help BUT respond (when you have one person who is agitated you have 2 and 3 and 4 etc..)

_____**Privacy** – forgetting to provide privacy

_____**Other**_____

G. DEVELOPING THE PLAN OF CARE

REMEMBER TO USE THE INFORMATION GATHERED FROM THE BEHAVIOUR MONITORING AND GRAPHING TOOLS

- **BRAINSTORM** with every person on the unit who has contact with the client using the information gathered through assessment and monitoring.
- Come to a **CONSESUS** regarding the behaviour to be targeted and the strategies to be utilized.
- **TARGET** only one behaviour at a time.
- **COMMUNICATE** the plan of care and intervention strategies to ensure a **CONSISTENT** approach by all staff.
- Set up time frames to **EVALUATE** the interventions.

BEHAVIOUR TO BE TARGETED:
_____
_____
_____

STRATEGY #1   Date initiated_____   Evaluation Date_____
_____
_____
_____

Results of evaluation _____
_____
_____

STRATEGY #2   Date initiated_____   Evaluation Date_____
_____
_____

Results of evaluation _____
_____
_____
_____

STRATEGY #3   Date initiated_____Evaluation Date_____
_____
_____

Results of evaluation_____
_____
_____
_____

Scientific Publishing House

offers

free of charge publication

of current academic research papers, Bachelor´s Theses, Master's Theses, Dissertations or Scientific Monographs

If you have written a thesis which satisfies high content as well as formal demands, and you are interested in a remunerated publication of your work, please send an e-mail with some initial information about yourself and your work to *info@vdm-publishing-house.com.*

Our editorial office will get in touch with you shortly.

VDM Publishing House Ltd.
Meldrum Court 17.
Beau Bassin
Mauritius
www.vdm-publishing-house.com

 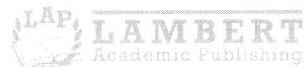 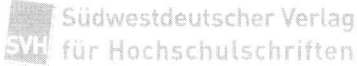

Printed in Great Britain by
Amazon.co.uk, Ltd.,
Marston Gate.